¡SALUD! VEGAN MEXICAN COOKBOOK

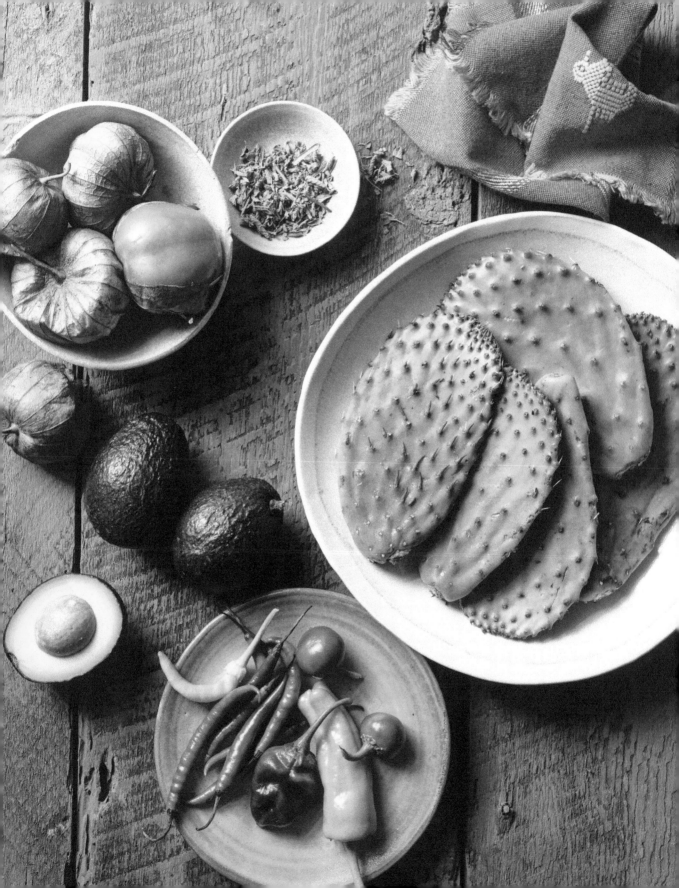

¡Salud!

VEGAN MEXICAN COOKBOOK

150 Mouthwatering Recipes from Tamales to Churros

EDDIE GARZA

Photography by Melina Hammer

ROCKRIDGE
PRESS

Photography © 2016 Melina Hammer
Author photo © Sylvia Elzafon

ISBN: Print 978-1-62315-778-4 | eBook 978-1-62315-779-1

Esto es para ti, Grandma.

(This is for you, Grandma.)

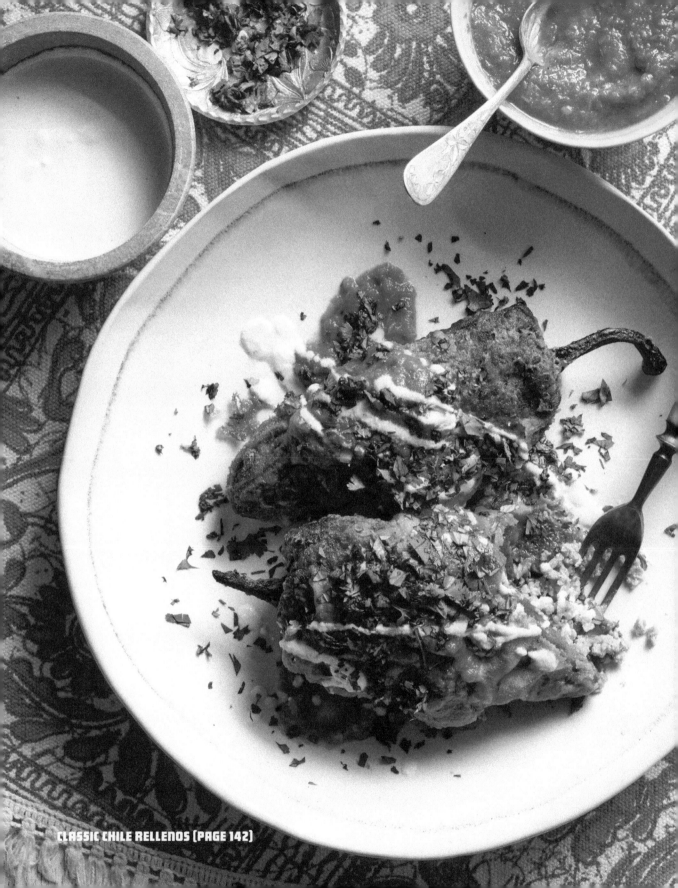

CLASSIC CHILE RELLENOS (PAGE 142)

Contents

Introduction

For as long as I can remember, I've been passionate about cooking. It's always played a major role in my life. My mother likes to tell the stories about how I made her breakfast-in-bed crepes when I was seven years old as a "get well" gesture, and how I baked a three-tier cake for my own 10th birthday. She always seems to leave out the part about how my cake turned out lopsided and flat. Truth is, it wasn't until after I learned a few things working at Spiral Diner, an all-vegan restaurant and bakery in Dallas, that I got my baking chops down.

I was born and raised in the South Texas border town of Brownsville by Mexican immigrant parents and an *abuelita* who taught me everything in the kitchen. My grandmother came to the United States from Guanajuato— arguably the most beautiful state in all of Mexico—and brought with her many wonderful traditions and food rituals, like communal cooking.

From an early age, I learned how to make Mexican staples like homemade corn and flour tortillas, beans *a la charra*, and Mexican red rice. I was also taught more elaborate pre-Hispanic foods like tamales, many of which we gave away as Christmas presents to friends and family. In fact, I still vividly remember making the rounds every Christmas eve to all my *tías'* and *tíos'* houses to proudly hand-deliver their dozens of tamales that took us all day to make.

Spending my childhood in the kitchen with Grandma was exciting and incredibly enriching. From her, I learned to embrace my mestizo heritage and celebrate the joys of Mexican cooking.

Mexico has a rich and diverse food history. In pre-Hispanic Mesoamerican cuisine, there was a big focus on fruits, vegetables, legumes, and grains. Grandma simplifies it: "Before the Spanish came to Mexico, food was provided by the sun and earth." My Spanish ancestors fused their culinary traditions with indigenous foods to shape modern Mexican cuisine.

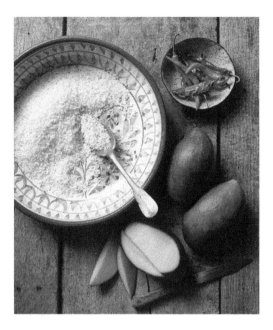

In the ancient Maya civilization, growing plants for food was so vital that the vast majority of the people were involved in vegetable farming; developing sophisticated systems to maximize production of beans, squash, and maize. Yum-Kaax—the Young Maize God—was perhaps the most important of the Maya deities, and is often depicted in Maya mythology wearing a headpiece in the shape of an ear of maize. Maize, just like rice in most East Asian countries and wheat in Europe, was the grain that served as the base for virtually every meal for the Maya.

The Aztec civilization used Maya staples like beans and corn, and also cultivated other crops like chile peppers, sweet potatoes, jicama, nopal cactus, peanuts, and grains like amaranth. The Aztec also grew an assortment of fruits, including tomatoes, guavas, papayas, and chirimoyas—which Mark Twain called "the most delicious fruit known to man."

When the Spanish settled in Mexico in the 1500s, their main contributions to food culture were meat and dairy products. They also introduced different cooking techniques, including frying foods in pork fat. Today's Mexican cuisine, the fusion of Mesoamerican and European cooking, is now notoriously known for its excessive use of meat, lard, and other animal products that have been linked to chronic, preventable diseases caused by obesity, such as type 2 diabetes, heart disease, and stroke.

In recent years, there's been a social gastronomic movement in Mexico focusing on indigenous foods, like legumes and grains, to combat the country's obesity epidemic. It's the momentum of this movement and my deep love for the kitchen that have made it such a joy to help take all Mexican food—from pre-Hispanic Mesoamerican to modern Mexican cuisine—back to its plant-centric roots. *¡Buen provecho!*

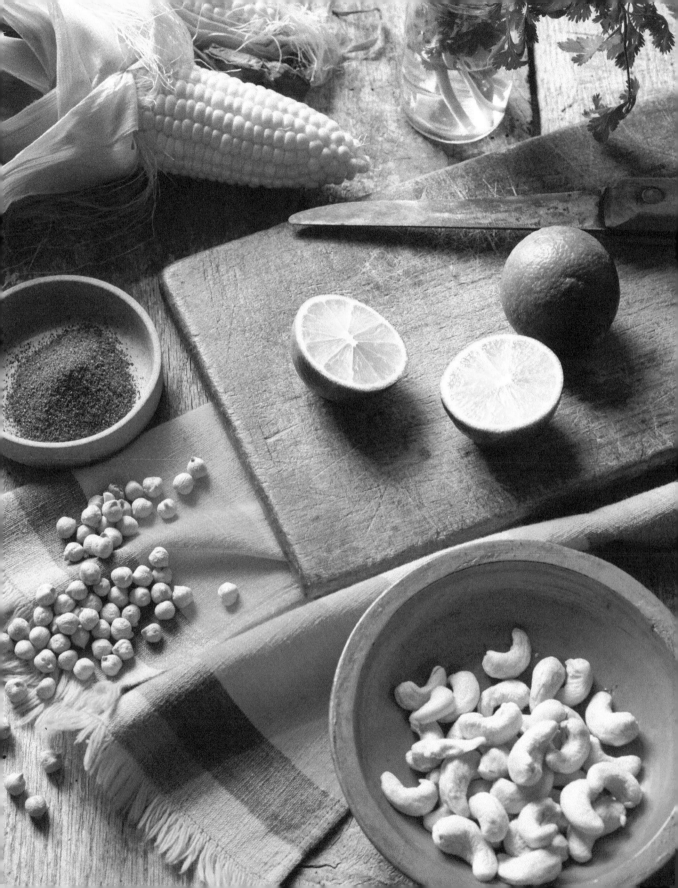

Chapter 1

LA COCINA VEGANA

Before the introduction of beef, pork, chicken, and dairy by Spanish conquistadores, the staples of Mexico were maize, chiles, potatoes, squashes, and other native fruits and vegetables—local food grown by indigenous people. But when most of us think of plant-based cooking, we think of bland cooking, not the complex, hearty flavors of modern Latin American cuisine.

¡Salud! Vegan Mexican Cookbook brings Mexican cuisine back to its healthy, pre-Hispanic plant-based roots without losing any of the favorite modern recipes, like guacamole and quesadillas. In addition, *¡Salud! Vegan Mexican Cookbook* introduces exciting new recipes like Cashew Queso Fundido (page 74) and Garbanzorizo (page 242). This cookbook is crammed full of fresh, approachable takes on familiar dishes and new favorites, from Chili sin Queso (page 75) to Aztec Spiced Pumpkin Soup (page 60), and straightforward swap-outs that bring fresh, wholesome foods back to the center of the plate—you'll realize that cooking well-balanced Mexican food without animal products is not only incredibly simple but *riquísimo* (delicious!) too.

SIN CARNE, SIN LECHE, SIN HUEVOS

By learning just a few basic techniques with these meat-free, egg-free, and dairy-free ingredients, you'll expand your palate and your pantry—proving you don't need any animal products to whip up delicious and nutritious Mexican meals.

MEATLESS MEXICAN

Tofu—Tofu is a versatile soy-based alternative for chicken, beef, and pork that readily absorbs any flavor. It comes in a remarkable variety of forms and textures, ranging from extra soft, to medium, to extra firm. Extra-firm tofu is perfect for cubing or slicing, and can be baked, grilled, fried, or even crumbled like ground meat. Firm tofu holds up well to pan frying or can be crumbled into a delicious tofu scramble. You can find tofu in most well-stocked grocery stores, although Asian markets and health food stores tend to carry a wider assortment of brands and forms to choose from.

Jackfruit—More commonly known as "vegan pulled pork" in the US, due to its remarkably meaty texture, jackfruit can be found fresh, canned, frozen, and preshredded in most Asian markets and some well-stocked health food stores. High in fiber and potassium, jackfruit is a fat-free, low-calorie alternative to pork, and its naturally mild flavor makes it a versatile ingredient that easily absorbs the flavors of practically any recipe—like my delicious Jackfruit Carnitas Tortas (page 99).

Textured vegetable protein (TVP)—TVP is a highly nutritious soy-based product that's super simple to cook and makes for perfect "ground beef" in practically any dish, like my Chili sin Carne (page 65) or Picadillo (page 63). The best part? You can find TVP in the produce section of most Latin markets.

Soy chorizo—Made with soy protein and the same spices as regular chorizo, soy chorizo is just as flavorful as the pork varieties, but a much healthier alternative, with less fat and zero cholesterol. Garbanzorizo (page 242) is a delicious, homemade vegan (and gluten-free) recipe for a mouthwatering chickpea version of this spicy Mexican sausage.

Seitan—With one of the meatiest textures, and packed with protein, seitan is an excellent meat alternative that I use in all my steak-style tacos and tortas—and marinate in chiles and pineapple for my Lebanese-Mexican fusion Tacos al Pastor (page 89). Made by processing vital wheat gluten, the natural protein found in wheat, seitan is strong enough to hold up to practically any style of cooking, from braising to grilling to frying. Vital wheat gluten is sold as a powder, and can be found in the baking section of any health food store and most well-stocked supermarkets. You can make delicious seasoned seitan at home (Mexican Seasoned Seitan, page 239), or buy it premade in most well-stocked grocery stores and any health food market.

Mushrooms—Packed with rich, deep, savory flavor, mushrooms are a simple and all-natural meat alternative. There's a wide variety of mushrooms to choose from: from easy-to-find white button mushrooms, perfect for swapping out pork or beef; to meaty oyster mushrooms as an alternative to chicken, as in my Chicken-Style Setas Tacos (page 95) and Aztec Seared Chicken-Style Setas Salad (page 51). They're wonderful in practically every recipe.

Eggplant—The bulk and texture of eggplant makes it a delicious and filling meat alternative in many dishes. Virtually fat-free and packed with essential vitamins and minerals, like potassium and vitamin C, eggplant is a high-fiber natural ingredient that goes great diced and tossed in a tofu scramble, or shredded and marinated for my ranch-style Spicy Eggplant Barbacoa Tacos (page 94).

Packaged vegan meats—A shortcut to capturing all of those savory flavors of pork, seafood, chicken, and beef, prepackaged vegan meat alternatives are a simple and convenient choice for cooks in a crunch. There are countless brands to choose from in most well-stocked grocery and health food stores, so no matter whether you're looking for the perfect meatless beefy crumbles or fish-free fillets, there's always a time-saving option out there for you.

SIN SEAFOOD

With so many kinds of fish and shellfish in so many different Mexican recipes, here are a few simple tips to help you replicate those distinctive tastes and textures.

Dulse flakes—A nutritious red seaweed, dulse can be found dried in most health food stores, and adds a savory sea-like flavor to any "seafood" dish.

Palm or artichoke hearts—With a toothsome texture similar to that of shellfish, palm and artichoke hearts have a mild flavor that works well in dishes like ceviche or my Seven Seas Soup (page 58).

Garbanzo beans—Also known as chickpeas, garbanzo beans are a high-protein, versatile legume that, when mashed, replicate the texture of fish in my delicious and filling Seafood-Style Albondigas (page 81).

Cauliflower—Beer-battered and fried, cauliflower makes a perfect stand-in for fish in my recipe for Baja Tacos (page 92).

LEAVING LECHE

If gooey enchiladas covered in cheese and dolloped with sour cream are the first dish that pops to mind, don't worry. There are ample nondairy options for creating stellar Mexican dishes.

Vegan sour cream—Delicious coconut, almond, and soy-based sour creams are all great dairy-free alternatives to traditional varieties. They can usually be found in your local health food store. Make sure to check the label, though, because some dairy-free sour creams still contain animal products, like whey or casein.

Vegan butter and margarine—Vegan butters are generally blends of water, plant-based fats, and flavorings to replicate the taste and texture of dairy-based butter. Common ingredients include coconut oil, cocoa butter, olive oil, nondairy milks like soy or coconut, and lecithin—but the selection has widened online in recent years to include even banana-based, garlic-based, and miso-tahini–based butters, among many others. If you can't find vegan butter in stores or online, consider using onion butter or mashed avocado—two easy at-home alternatives.

> *Onion butter*—Chopped and sautéed, onions can be simmered for several hours in just enough water to cover them until they become sweet and dark-brown, and easily spreadable. When cool, this creamy onion butter can be served immediately, or frozen or refrigerated for later use.

> *Mashed avocado*—Simply mashing a ripe avocado—naturally filled with healthy monounsaturated fats—yields a spreadable butter that can also take the place of dairy-based butter in many baking recipes.

Vegan cheese—Made from various plant proteins, from soy to safflower, tapioca, and nuts, there are numerous brands of vegan cheeses available at most health food stores and well-stocked grocery stores, as well as a handful of recipes here to make at home, like Almond Queso Cotija (page 73) and Cashew Queso Fundido (page 74). Depending on the process and ingredients, vegan cheeses can vary widely in taste and texture—just like dairy-based cheese—a perfect excuse to try a number of popular brands to find which ones best suit your taste.

Vegan cream cheese—A creamy plant-based ingredient I use in my Picadillo Empanadas (page 104), vegan cream cheese is a delicious, dairy-free alternative that can be found in most health food stores and well-stocked grocery stores. Both soy-based and almond-based versions work wonderfully.

Cashew milk—Cashew milk, made from water and blended cashews, is a great source of antioxidants and fiber. Creamy cashew milk can be found at any well-stocked grocery store or bodega.

Cashew cream—A thicker, nuttier variation of cashew milk, cashew cream can be used in both savory and sweet vegan dishes, from sour "cream" to top your tacos or nacho "cheese," to vegan ice creams and other succulent desserts. I use it as the cream base for Seitan Enchiladas Suizas (page 154) and as a garnish for my Burritos Enmolados (page 130).

Soymilk—Soymilk is the most widely accessible of the common dairy-free milks. Naturally high in protein, soymilk can be found in nearly all well-stocked grocery stores or bodegas.

Rice milk—Made from the natural starches of boiled brown rice, rice milk holds up best to heat among the dairy-free milk options, making it wonderful for baking. But perhaps the best way to enjoy this nut-free milk is in my spiced Horchata Mexicana (page 213).

Almond milk—Almond milk is a simple, low-fat choice that's naturally high in vitamin E, selenium, iron, and potassium. Almond milk is a delicious alternative to cow's milk that is simple enough to make at home, but can also be found in most well-stocked grocery stores and bodegas. Its creaminess and versatility make it the perfect nut milk for my Café sin Leche (page 211).

Nutritional yeast—Nutritional yeast, also known as "nooch," is a dairy-free, gluten-free alternative to cheese, with an unmistakably delicious cheesy flavor that can easily replace Parmesan and other aged cheeses. Nutritional yeast is inactivated, meaning it does not froth or leaven like baking yeast, and is usually packed with protein, folic acid, and vitamin B_{12}—making it a great addition to any diet. Nutritional yeast enhances vegan cheese sauces like my Chili sin Queso (page 75), gives an eggy flavor to egg-free scrambles, and adds depth to any recipe. In recipes where nutritional yeast is used for its cheesy flavor, it is best not to substitute anything else, but small amounts of miso or soy sauce may add a similar rich and savory flavor. Nutritional yeast can be found both powdered and flaked online, in the natural food aisle of well-stocked supermarkets, or at your local health food or vitamin store.

HASTA HUEVOS

Wondering how we're going to make *migas sin huevos*? Here are a few of my favorite subs.

Silken tofu—This Japanese variety of tofu has a creamy custard texture, and generally can be found either soft, firm, or extra firm. While firm tofu makes an excellent vegan egg alternative when crumbled (Tofu Huevos, page 237), firm silken tofu is the perfect match for slightly runny eggs (Tofu Huevos Rancheros, page 35).

Vegan mayo—Made with vegetable oils, water, emulsifiers, and other flavorings to mimic the texture and taste of egg-based mayonnaise, vegan mayo is available in most health food stores and can replace eggs as a binding agent, as in my Mexican Chocolate Cake (page 218). My preferred brand is Just Mayo by Hampton Creek, which is available at most major supermarkets. While you're shopping for vegan mayo, pick up a vegan chipotle mayo as well. It makes a great spread for tortas.

Flax meal—Another excellent binder, flax meal can be found in most health food stores and also replaces eggs in some vegan recipes, like my Black Bean Burguesa Tortas (page 100).

Aquafaba—From the Latin words for "water" and "bean," aquafaba is the brine from canned chickpeas. When whisked together with a little flour, it makes the perfect egg-free batter for Classic Chile Rellenos (page 142). You can also use aquafaba to make meringue toppings and most baked goods that traditionally call for eggs.

Egg-replacement products—There are numerous vegan "faux egg" products on the shelves of well-stocked grocery stores that are an excellent, easy-to-find alternative to eggs in most baking recipes. Follow Your Heart makes a soy-free, gluten-free, nut-free egg replacer.

CON SABOR

Why does Mexican food taste so great? Now that we've gone through staples for a well-stocked vegan kitchen, let's explore the flavorful (and potentially unfamiliar) ingredients you'll need for your Mexican *cocina vegana*.

Achiote—Also known as annatto, achiote is a spice with a subtle, earthy flavor, and can generally be found in Oaxacan and Yucatán cuisine. Ground with garlic, lime juice, and spices such as cumin, cloves, and Mexican oregano, achiote paste makes a zesty addition to tamales or empanada dough. Achiote can be found online, in your local Latin market, or the international aisle of most grocery stores. Substitutes for achiote include turmeric, paprika, and nutmeg.

Amaranth—Grown and revered by the Aztecs before the arrival of the Spanish, amaranth grain is gluten-free, remarkably versatile, and high in protein and fiber. Amaranth adds a nutty flavor and texture to breads, hot cereals, and granolas, as in my Amaranth Granola with Oats and Mexican Chocolate (page 32). While it's sold in most well-stocked grocery stores, if you can't find amaranth, both quinoa and millet are acceptable substitutes in many recipes.

Avocado—Native to Mexico, the avocado is a creamy fruit full of healthy monounsaturated fats. A ripe avocado is slightly soft when gently squeezed, and usually served raw as a guacamole base or simply spread on tortillas. The most common variety found in the US is the smaller, purple-black Hass, although the nuttier, green-skinned Fuerte avocados are popular in much of Southern California. Avocados can be found at most grocery stores.

Banana leaves—Banana leaves are another choice for tamales, and are used in the more tropical and southern regions of Mexico, as in the popular Oaxacan style. Often wilted before use, fresh banana leaves can be found in most Asian or Latin markets. Compared to cornhusks, banana leaves infuse a subtle, sweet flavor and tend to result in wetter masa (also called masa harina or corn flour) when steamed.

Bolillo—Brought to Mexico City in the mid-19th century, the bolillo is a white bread similar to a French baguette, but shorter and wider, with a crunchy crust, soft interior, and distinctive oblong shape. It's an essential ingredient to any torta (sandwich) or mollete (bread topped with beans, salsa, and cheese). Bolillos are best eaten fresh and quickly go stale. If you cannot find them at your local *panadería* (Latin bakery), a baguette or hoagie roll may be a good substitute.

Chirimoya—Also known as custard apple or ice cream fruit, the chirimoya—sometimes spelled *cherimoya*—is well known for its delicious, creamy flesh. With a tropical flavor described as similar to coconut, strawberry, pineapple, banana, and papaya, chirimoya can be best appreciated in ice creams and smoothies, or simply chilled and eaten with a spoon. Chirimoya can be found in most Asian markets, or substitute a mixture of banana, pineapple, and strawberry in many recipes.

Cilantro—With its fresh, distinct flavor, cilantro is a versatile herb found in most grocery stores that is an essential ingredient in many Mexican dishes. However, a small percentage of people perceive cilantro as having an overwhelming soapy taste—making for an occasionally divisive ingredient at the dinner table. If this sounds like you, consider substituting parsley or celery leaf.

Cinnamon—With a unique, sweet-spicy flavor, cinnamon is a popular and versatile spice in Mexican cuisine, found in both savory and sweet dishes—and is a key ingredient in my Aztec Spice Blend (page 229). Cinnamon can be found in most grocery stores.

Corn/maize—A staple crop for over 10,000 years in Mexico, maize has been at the very heart of Mexican cuisine since the rise of the ancient Maya people. From elotes (corn on the cob) to tamales, corn is a versatile ingredient that can be found in both contemporary and pre-Hispanic Mexican dishes, from simple preparations to elaborate recipes, fresh or nixtimalized (treated with lime) and ground to masa flour. Cornmeal is simply finely ground dried corn, and is not the same as masa; neither is yellow corn grits, a coarser grind of corn. Masa, also called masa harina, is corn flour. Find fresh corn at your local farmers' market or grocery store, and masa flour at most Latin markets and supermarkets.

Cornhusks—Cornhusks are common wrappers for Mexican-style steamed tamales. Purchased in most Latin markets, dried cornhusks should be soaked in warm water before use, until they are soft and pliable. Cornhusks have a rough side and smooth side; for easy unwrapping, always spread the masa (tamale dough) on the smooth side of the husks. Cornhusk tamales tend to be firmer than those steamed in banana leaves, imparting an additional depth to the masa's corn flavor.

Cumin—Found in Latin American, South Asian, and North African cooking, iron-rich cumin has a distinctive earthy flavor. A warm addition to any soup or stew, cumin can be bought ground or as whole seeds at most well-stocked grocery stores.

Dulse—Dulse is a nutrient-dense red seaweed that grows wild along the Atlantic and Pacific Coasts. More densely packed with vitamins and minerals than kale or spinach, dulse is also a great source of protein and natural fiber—and adds a savory punch to any dish. Once harvested, dulse is typically dried, and can be found online or in well-stocked grocery stores in powder, flake, and whole-leaf varieties. If you can't find dulse, try nori, kelp, or wakame.

Epazote—Also known as Mexican tea, epazote has a distinctive, pungent flavor. Commonly cooked with black beans or brewed into teas, epazote may be found fresh or dried at most Mexican specialty stores and is found in a variety of Mexican dishes. While no other herb quite captures epazote's unique flavor, cilantro or parsley may be added to recipes in its place.

Hearts of palm—Harvested from the inner core of the stems of certain palm trees, palm hearts have a crisp texture and flavor, similar to artichoke hearts. Palm hearts are found canned in most grocery stores and may be served in many recipes, especially salads and soups. Artichoke hearts or water chestnut are good substitutes.

Hominy—Hominy are nixtamalized maize kernels, or corn, soaked in an alkaline solution to remove the hull and improve the nutritional content. Traditionally found in menudo (spice tripe soup) and pozole (hominy stew), these kernels are about three times the size of raw corn kernels, with a chewy texture and an unmistakable nutty-corn flavor. They can be found canned or dried at most well-stocked grocery stores. In soups or stews, dried beans are acceptable substitutes.

Huitlachoche—Also known as the corn truffle or corn mushroom, huitlacoche is a traditional Mexican delicacy with a smoky, earthy flavor that can be used in any dish where you might use a mushroom, from tamales to quesadillas. Huitlacoche is a highly sought-after ingredient, increasingly popular in fine dining. It can be found canned in most Latin grocery stores and at well-stocked farmers' markets.

Jicama—A large root vegetable native to Central America, jicama has a slightly sweet flavor and white, crunchy flesh similar to an apple. In fact, you can substitute apples for jicama in many recipes. Although edible, the skin is fibrous and is usually removed. Jicama can be sliced and served raw, or cooked similar to a potato. When cooked gently, water chestnuts are a better substitute. Look for jicama in the produce sections of supermarkets and specialty stores.

Mexican chocolate—This form of chocolate is meant for cooking rather than nibbling for dessert. Compared to other varieties of chocolate, Mexican chocolate tends to have a less-processed, grainer texture and a deeper, spicier flavor—and can be found in a wide range of traditional Mexican dishes, from hot chocolate to Brown Mole (page 196). Mexican chocolate can be found in most Latin grocery stores.

Mexican oregano—Native to Central and South America, Mexican oregano has a more complex, citrusy flavor than Mediterranean oregano. It pairs deliciously with tomatillos, chiles, and other common Mexican ingredients. Mexican oregano can be found fresh or dried in most Latin grocery stores, or you can substitute the Mediterranean variety.

Nopales—Commonly known in the US as prickly pear cactus, nopales are usually sold fresh and cleaned of spines in Hispanic specialty stores, but may also be found canned or jarred in grocery stores. Nopales are a popular Mexican ingredient in tacos, salads, or served on their own. They have a crisp, slightly tart flavor. Green beans may be substituted in most recipes, although they lack nopales' characteristic "slick" texture.

Pepitas— These unsalted, hulled, roasted pumpkin seeds are a popular ingredient in Mexico and the US, and are commonly found in a number of traditional recipes. Serve pepitas as a topper on any salad—or simply spice and roast them for a simple and delicious snack, such as Aztec Spiced Pepitas (page 69). Buy pepitas in any well-stocked grocery store. If you can't find pepitas, try unsalted sunflower seeds or pistachios.

Piloncillo—Minimally processed cane sugar, piloncillo usually comes in a solid cone and has an earthy, rum-like, caramel taste. Used in both savory and sweet recipes, piloncillo complements the flavors of fruits, beans, and dried chiles, and deepens the flavor of any dessert. It must be broken into small pieces to cook with it. Use a sharp, serrated knife to scrape and chop it off the cone. Or for very fine piloncillo, use a box grater. If the piloncillo is very hard, you can microwave it for 10 or 20 seconds to soften it before chopping. Piloncillo is easily found in most Hispanic grocery stores, but you can substitute dark brown sugar. Lighter varieties have a milder flavor than darker piloncillos.

Radish—A garnish on many Mexican dishes since its introduction to Mexican cuisine by the Spanish, sliced radish adds a fresh, peppery bite and pop of color to tacos and sopas. Consider using jicama and lime for a similar effect. Radishes can be found in most well-stocked grocery stores.

Squash/zucchini blossoms—Found in summer and early fall, squash blossoms have a fresh, floral, zucchini flavor, and a surprisingly hearty texture—making them popular for stuffing or frying, or as the star of Zucchini Blossom Quesadillas (page 78). You can also eat them raw. Find them in the spring and summer at most farmers' markets. Unsprayed day lilies are an acceptable substitute in most recipes.

Tomatillo—A close relative of the tomato, the tomatillo is a Mexican staple with a tart flavor and green flesh that is found in many green salsas, including Roasted Tomatillo Salsa (page 201). They're found fresh or canned in most Latin markets—remove the papery hull from the fresh ones. You can substitute green (underripe) tomatoes sprinkled with lime juice.

CHILES

Chiles are an essential ingredient for any Mexican kitchen. But not all chiles are created equal. Some are sweet, some are spicy, and they come in a variety of forms, from fresh to dried to powdered. Many of the recipes in this book call for dried chiles that are reconstituted and made into pastes to create a base. Here are the most common chiles used in Mexican cuisine.

Ancho—When the poblano chile is dried, it becomes flat, sweet, and wrinkled and is known as chile ancho. A staple of Mexican dishes like tamales, for most recipes ancho chiles must be soaked and rehydrated before use. Anchos can be found in most Latin markets. You can substitute poblanos, along with ½ teaspoon of liquid smoke, per pepper.

Chiles de árbol—Also known as the bird's beak chile, chiles de árbol can be found fresh, dried, or powdered online and at most Latin markets. A small, red, and powerfully spicy chile native to Mexico, powdered chile de árbol may be replaced with cayenne pepper, or when fresh, with pequin chiles.

Chipotle—Chipotle chiles have a similar level of heat as fresh jalapeños. Dried or canned in adobo sauce, chipotle chiles can be found in most Latin markets; you can substitute chipotle powder, found in most well-stocked

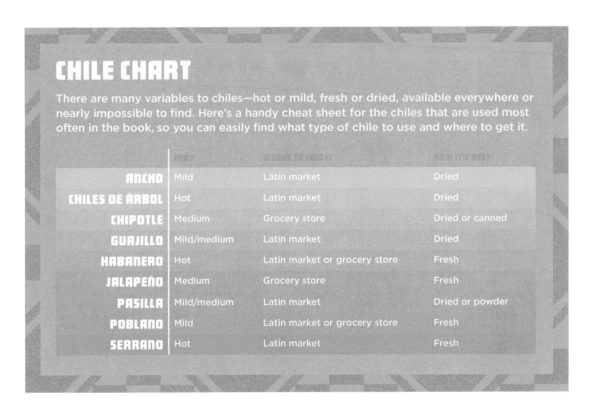

CHILE CHART

There are many variables to chiles—hot or mild, fresh or dried, available everywhere or nearly impossible to find. Here's a handy cheat sheet for the chiles that are used most often in the book, so you can easily find what type of chile to use and where to get it.

	HEAT	WHERE TO FIND IT	HOW IT'S BEST
ANCHO	Mild	Latin market	Dried
CHILES DE ÁRBOL	Hot	Latin market	Dried
CHIPOTLE	Medium	Grocery store	Dried or canned
GUAJILLO	Mild/medium	Latin market	Dried
HABANERO	Hot	Latin market or grocery store	Fresh
JALAPEÑO	Medium	Grocery store	Fresh
PASILLA	Mild/medium	Latin market	Dried or powder
POBLANO	Mild	Latin market or grocery store	Fresh
SERRANO	Hot	Latin market	Fresh

grocery stores. You can replace them with jalepeños, along with ½ teaspoon of liquid smoke, per chile. Typically, I use both the chile and some of the sauce in the can.

Guajillo—The guajillo (the dried version of the Mirasol chile) is a mild to medium hot chile that is second only to the ancho in popularity in Mexico. Guajillo, which means "little gourd," got its name for the rattling sound of the seeds within the dried chile pods. The guajillo is a key ingredient for Classic Chile Paste (page 194), and adds a little bit of heat and color to Black Bean Tamales (page 108) and Arroz Enchilado (page 164). You can find this popular dried chile at any Latin market or well-stocked grocer.

Habanero—A very hot spicy chile with citrusy notes, habaneros are small and orange or red when ripe. An important ingredient in much of the cuisine in the Yucatan region of Mexico, habaneros are commonly found in many hot sauce recipes. Scotch bonnet chiles can replace habaneros in most recipes— or use jalapeños and double the number of chiles.

Jalapeño—Jalapeño chiles are green, with a medium heat level. A versatile chile, jalapeños can be found in most grocery stores fresh or pickled, and are found in any number of popular Mexican dishes, from salsas to salads, charred or stuffed. Or they can simply be sliced and used as a fresh and spicy garnish. You can substitute serrano chiles, but halve the number of chiles used.

Pasilla—Named for its dark, wrinkled skin that resembles a small raisin, the pasilla is a mild to medium chile that is the dried form of the chilaco chile. Pasillas are richly flavored chiles, so they work wonderfully in moles and salsas, including my Brown Mole (page 196) and Chiles de Árbol Salsa (page 203). Pasillas can be found at any Latin market in whole or powdered form.

Poblano—A large, mild green chile, the poblano can be found in popular dishes like Classic Chile Rellenos (page 142)—or covered in walnut sauce and topped with pomegranate seeds to replicate the colors of the Mexican flag in the traditional Independence Day dish Chiles en Nogada (page 146). The poblano can be found in most grocery stores in the American Southwest and in any Latin market.

Serrano—Serrano chiles are small, pointed, very hot chiles native to the Mexican states of Pueblo and Hidalgo. One of the most popular chiles in Mexican cuisine, the serrano chile can add a kick of heat to any recipe. You can find serranos fresh at most Latin markets, and in the produce section of many well-stocked grocery stores. Habaneros and jalapeños are acceptable substitutes.

COOKING TOOLS

Mexican cuisine is a complex combination of ingredients and techniques. And as in many of the cuisines from around the globe, culinary traditions and techniques have been passed from generation to generation—oftentimes without an actual recipe—meaning that having the right tools can make a real difference in your meals.

Molcajete—A pre-Hispanic stone grinding bowl similar to the mortar and pestle, the molcajete (mortar) and tejolote (pestle) are traditionally carved from basalt. Molcajetes are often used to grind spices and to prepare salsas and guacamoles. You need to season your new molcajete by grinding handfuls of rice in it until no grains of basalt are visible. With use, it will "season" like quality cast iron.

Tortilla press—Tortilla presses, or tortilleras, are modern tools used to simplify the preparation of thin, round handmade corn tortillas. You simply put a ball of dough in and press. Commonly found in aluminum, wood, or cast iron, the cast-iron varieties tend to hold up best to repeated use. Electric gadgets are sold that press and cook tortillas—but the cheaper, human-powered presses are just as convenient. A tortilla press is nice to have because it makes tortilla prep fast and easy, but you can also use a rolling pin to press tortillas if you aren't *pressed* for time.

Rolling pin—Used to prepare Handmade Flour Tortillas (page 233) and empanadas, wooden rolling pins are one of a number of simple tools you can use to work with dough. Buy rolling pins at any cookware store, Latin market, or well-stocked grocery store.

Tamal steamer—In most Latin markets, you can find tamal steamers in a variety of sizes, from 12 to 32 quarts. They are usually made from aluminum, enamel, or stainless steel. Buy whichever kind fits your budget, but make sure it is at least a 16-quart steamer to comfortably accommodate all the varieties of tamales featured in this book. If you can't find a tamal steamer, or don't have the kitchen space to store another large pot, you can use a stock pot with a tight lid and a steamer insert, or a stovetop-safe roasting pan covered with aluminum foil.

Comal—A versatile flat cast-iron griddle commonly found in Mexican and Central American kitchens, the comal is often used to cook tortillas, vegetables, chiles, and any number of other foods. A quality comal becomes seasoned over time, like any other cast-iron pan. You can find one at any Latin market or online; if you already have a flat cast-iron pancake griddle, that will serve the purpose.

A WORD ABOUT LABELS

You will find the following labels used in the recipes in this book.

SOY-FREE

NUT-FREE

GLUTEN-FREE

QUICK & EASY

Quick & Easy means the whole dish, from prep to table, takes 30 minutes or less. Recipes that require you to make component recipes will not be labeled Quick & Easy unless the complete total time is less than 30 minutes.

As for the other labels, when working with vegan alternatives, things are not always straightforward. Some vegan dairy alternatives, for example, have soy or nuts and some do not. I use Daiya or Follow Your Heart brands of vegan sour cream, butter, margarine, shredded cheese, and cream cheese because they are all nut-free, soy-free, and gluten-free.

However, just to be cautious, I've assumed the products listed here have the common allergens listed with them. Some things can't be avoided (tofu, tempeh, and TVP will always have soy, for example, and seitan will always have gluten), but many of the recipes that are not labeled nut-free or soy-free can be made so, simply by choosing your vegan dairy alternatives wisely. You'll notice that many of the recipes offer options for garnishes. I haven't included these garnishes in the labels (so, a recipe that lists optional cashew cream will be labeled nut-free, or one that calls for optional vegan cheese might have the soy-free label).

Tofu ....soy
Tempeh..soy
Textured vegetable protein (TVP).............soy
Seitan..gluten
Vegan sour cream...soy or nuts
Vegan butter or margarine........................soy
Vegan cheese...soy or nuts
Vegan cream cheese....................................soy or nuts

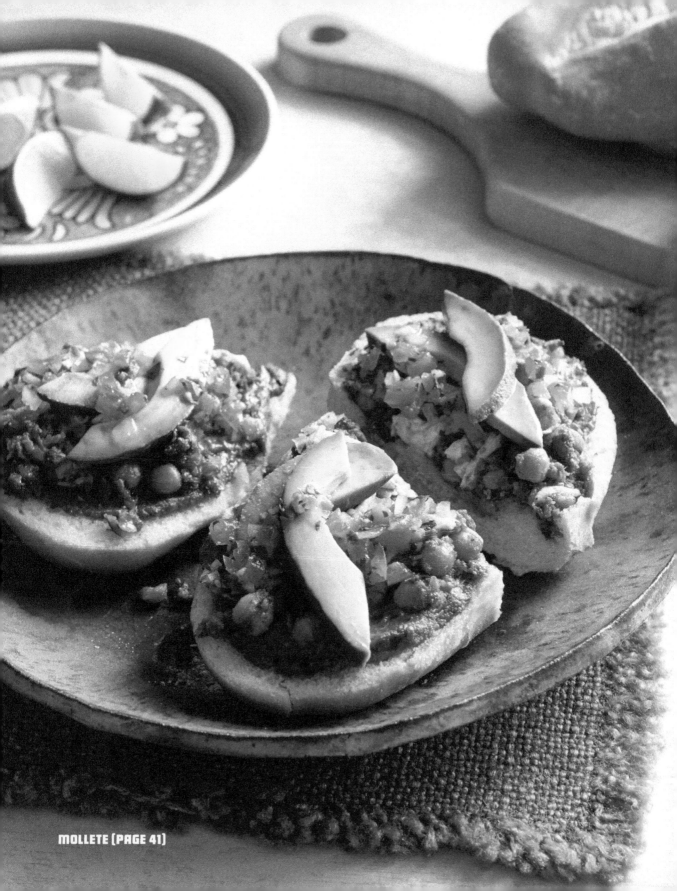

MOLLETE (PAGE 41)

Chapter 2

BREAKFAST

ARROZ SIN LECHE

SERVES 4 • PREP TIME: 5 MINUTES • COOK TIME: 30 MINUTES

While largely considered a dessert in Mexico, arroz con leche (Mexican rice pudding) has become a popular Mexican breakfast dish throughout Texas and the American Southwest. Variations of rice pudding can be found around the world. In Mexico, it's typically made with milk, cinnamon, sugar, vanilla, orange zest, and raisins. My Arroz sin Leche uses almond milk and piloncillo, an unrefined Mexican sugar made from pure cane. If you can't find piloncillo, simply replace it with equal amounts of dark brown sugar.

4 cups water
4 cinnamon sticks
2 cups white rice
2 cups unsweetened almond milk
1 to 2 teaspoons vanilla extract
½ teaspoon salt
3 tablespoons piloncillo

GARNISH OPTIONS
Raisins
Almonds
Toasted coconut shreds
Orange zest

1. Bring the water and cinnamon sticks to a boil in a large saucepan. Add the rice and lower the heat to a simmer. Cover and cook for 25 to 30 minutes.

2. Add the almond milk and turn the heat up to medium. Add the vanilla, salt, and piloncillo. Cook for 5 more minutes to thicken, stirring constantly to avoid burning the bottom. Reduce the heat, if necessary.

3. Portion into coffee cups or small bowls. Top with the garnishes of your choice and enjoy.

SIMPLE SWAP: Try replacing the almond milk with cashew milk or any other nut milk.

AMARANTH GRANOLA WITH OATS AND MEXICAN CHOCOLATE

MAKES 8 CUPS • PREP TIME: 10 MINUTES • COOK TIME: 30 MINUTES

Like maize, amaranth was a major crop of the Aztecs. In pre-Hispanic times, the grain was considered so sacred, it was often used in human sacrifices to honor the Aztec gods. When the Spanish arrived in Mexico, the cultivation of amaranth was banned because the Aztec ritual was condemned by the Catholic Church. Amaranth has made a big comeback recently because of its powerful health benefits, and the efforts of health and agriculture experts who've worked hard to bring this grain back to Mexico. My amaranth granola is a delicious mestizo marriage between popped amaranth and oats, which were brought to Mexico by the Spanish. They are blended with nuts, cinnamon, piloncillo, and spiced Mexican chocolate.

¾ cup vegan butter

2 teaspoons vanilla

½ teaspoon salt

1 tablespoon ground cinnamon

3 tablespoons piloncillo

3 ounces Mexican chocolate, divided

2 cups oats

2 cups popped amaranth

⅓ cup almonds

⅓ cup pepitas

½ cup raisins

½ cup unsweetened coconut flakes

1. Preheat the oven to 300°F and line a large baking sheet with parchment paper.

2. Put the butter, vanilla, salt, cinnamon, and piloncillo in a microwave-safe bowl and microwave for 1 minute, or until the piloncillo is dissolved. Add 1 ounce of chocolate and stir until smooth and well combined. Or on the stovetop, melt the butter in a small saucepan. With a potato peeler, shave in 1 ounce of chocolate as the butter melts. Add the vanilla, salt, cinnamon, and piloncillo. Remove from the heat.

3. In a large bowl, mix the oats, amaranth, almonds, and pepitas. Pour the hot melted butter mixture over the dry ingredients and combine. Spread the granola evenly onto the prepared baking sheet.

4. Bake for 20 to 30 minutes, stirring twice during cooking. While it's baking, chop the remaining 2 ounces of chocolate.

5. Remove the granola from the oven and let it cool completely. Mix in the raisins, coconut flakes, and remaining chocolate.

6. Amaranth granola keeps for 2 weeks in a sealed container.

SECRET INGREDIENT: Most Latin markets carry pre-popped amaranth. If there's no Latin market near you, don't worry! Just pop your own. Heat a skillet to high heat and add 1 teaspoon at a time of the raw grain to the heated pan. The amaranth will start popping within 2 to 3 seconds.

STONE-GROUND MAIZE MEAL PORRIDGE

SERVES 4 • PREP TIME: 10 • COOK TIME: 15 MINUTES

Cultivated in Mexico since early Maya times, maize is a versatile grain that takes on many shapes and forms in Mexican cuisine. One of my go-to breakfasts is this savory stone-ground maize meal seasoned with fresh cilantro, lime, and chile. It's just spicy enough to charge you up in the morning and hearty enough to keep you satisfied until lunchtime. You'll find roasted green chiles in cans in the grocery store.

1 small yellow onion, finely diced
1 tablespoon minced fresh garlic
¼ cup diced roasted green chiles from a jar
1 chipotle chile, chopped
2 cups Homemade Vegetable Stock (page 231), divided

1 tablespoon ground cumin
½ teaspoon salt
1 teaspoon freshly ground black pepper
½ cup yellow corn grits
3 tablespoons nutritional yeast
Juice of 1 lime
¼ cup chopped cilantro

1. In a large pan, sauté the onion, garlic, green chiles, and chipotle in 2 tablespoons of Homemade Vegetable Stock for about 7 minutes. Add the cumin, salt, pepper, and remaining Homemade Vegetable Stock and bring to a boil.

2. Whisk in the corn grits and cook on low heat 5 to 7 minutes.

3. Stir in the nutritional yeast, lime juice, and cilantro.

4. Adjust the seasonings and serve hot.

COOKING TIP: Use leftover maize meal porridge to make crispy maize cakes. Spread the meal 1 inch thick on a pan and refrigerate, then cut into 3-inch squares. Heat a skillet on medium-high heat and lightly oil the pan. Toast the squares until they're nicely golden brown on both sides. Top with some chili or a hearty soup, or just eat them all by themselves.

TOFU HUEVOS RANCHEROS

GF

NF

SERVES 4 • PREP TIME: 10 MINUTES • COOK TIME: 10 MINUTES

My father, who grew up on a farm in the northern state of Tamaulipas, used to make this classic breakfast dish with the eggs slightly runny, served over a single fried corn tortilla nestled in a spicy red ranchero sauce. This updated egg-free version calls for firm silken tofu to mimic slightly runny eggs, but the star remains Dad's spicy ranchero sauce and his perfect egg spice blend.

1 tablespoon olive oil
½ teaspoon garlic powder
½ teaspoon ground cumin
½ teaspoon chili powder
½ teaspoon freshly ground
   black pepper
Salt
1 (12-ounce) package silken tofu,
   crumbled into large chunks
1 cup Salsa Ranchera (page 199)

GARNISH OPTIONS
Chopped cilantro
Thinly sliced red onions
Squeeze of fresh lime juice

1. Heat a large skillet on medium-high heat. Add the oil, garlic powder, cumin, chili powder, and pepper, and season with salt. Sauté for 1 to 2 minutes. Add the tofu and cook until it is heated through. Or, for firmer tofu huevos, cook the tofu until it is slightly browned.

2. Add the Salsa Ranchera and heat through.

3. Serve hot, topped with the garnishes of your choice.

ORIGIN STORY: Huevos rancheros is a common breakfast in rural areas of northern Mexico. It has now spread throughout the Americas and has hundreds of variations.

POTATO, BLACK BEAN, AND TOFU HUEVO TAQUITOS

MAKES 8 TAQUITOS • PREP TIME: 20 • COOK TIME: 30 MINUTES

If there's one meal that takes me way back to childhood, it's papas con frijoles y tofu huevos—potato, bean, and tofu eggs. I have fond memories of helping Grandma peel potatoes on Saturday mornings while we watched Odisea Burbujas, *a Mexican TV show about crazy creatures and a wacky professor traveling through space. As the potatoes soaked, we'd sit at our avocado-green bar counter and laugh hysterically at Professor Memelovsky's follies. My* tía *Silvana used to top her potato taquitos with ketchup, which sounds strange, but it's actually pretty delicious. I like to go more traditional by topping mine with fresh avocado slices and salsa.*

1 large russet potato, peeled and diced into ½-inch cubes
1½ to 2 tablespoons canola oil
½ cup cooked black beans
1 cup Tofu Huevos (page 237)
1 teaspoon salt
¼ teaspoon freshly ground black pepper
¼ teaspoon garlic powder
8 corn tortillas

GARNISH OPTIONS
1 avocado, sliced
Roasted Tomatillo Salsa (page 201)

1. Soak the diced potatoes in cold water for 10 to 15 minutes to remove any extra starch, then drain.

2. Heat the oil in a large pan and cook the potatoes on medium heat for 20 minutes, covered. Stir occasionally.

3. Add the black beans, Tofu Huevos, salt, pepper, and garlic powder, and cook for 10 minutes, stirring halfway, to lightly brown evenly.

4. Serve hot with warm tortillas and the garnishes of your choice.

HEAT INDEX: To kick up the heat, toss a sliced and seeded jalapeño or serrano chile in with the potatoes halfway through sautéing.

VEGGIE CHORIZO WITH TOFU HUEVOS

SERVES 4 • PREP TIME: 5 MINUTES • COOK TIME: 15 MINUTES

Think of chorizo as you would bacon. It's so highly seasoned and intense in flavor, it's almost always used as an ingredient in Mexican cuisine. One of the most popular breakfasts throughout Mexico is chorizo con huevos—chorizo with scrambled eggs. Go to any authentic Mexican restaurant for breakfast—or any Mexican family's Sunday breakfast bonanza—and you're sure to find chorizo con huevos on the menu. This vegged-out version features my spicy Garbanzorizo and savory Tofu Huevos, which should both be staples in any vegan Mexican kitchen.

1 teaspoon canola oil
2 cups Tofu Huevos (page 237)
1 cup Garbanzorizo (page 242) or
    prepackaged seitan chorizo
2 tablespoons chopped cilantro
4 corn or 6-inch flour tortillas

GARNISH OPTIONS
Chunky Red Salsa (page 200)
Pico de Gallo (page 198)

1. In a large skillet, heat the oil and cook the Tofu Huevos for 10 minutes, stirring occasionally. Add the Garbanzorizo and cook for 5 to 7 minutes, stirring constantly. Add the cilantro and combine.

2. Serve hot with warm corn or flour tortillas and the garnishes of your choice.

SECRET INGREDIENT: Soy chorizo can be found in the tofu section of most grocery stores. Cook it in a separate skillet before adding to the tofu huevos. Once the chorizo and tofu huevos are combined, cook for 2 to 3 minutes before serving.

MIGAS

GF

NF

SERVES 4 • PREP TIME: 10 MINUTES • COOK TIME: 30 MINUTES

If there's one breakfast I ate more than any other as a kid, it's migas. Ask any Chicano who grew up on the border and you might get the same answer. Migas are traditionally made by lightly pan frying day-old tortillas and scrambling them up with eggs. For a lower-fat version, try oven-baking the tortillas. Simply spread cut tortilla squares evenly on a large baking sheet and bake at 350°F for 7 to 10 minutes.

8 corn tortillas
2½ tablespoons canola oil, divided
¼ medium yellow onion, julienned
1 poblano chile, seeded and julienned
1 Roma tomato, diced
2 cups Tofu Huevos (page 237)
Salt

GARNISH OPTIONS
Lime wedges
Pico de Gallo (page 198)

1. Cut the tortillas into 1-inch squares. Heat 2 tablespoons of oil in a large pan and toast the tortillas on medium-high heat, tossing the squares gently and constantly to prevent clumping. When they are slightly crispy but still tender, remove from the heat and set aside.

2. In a separate skillet, heat the remaining ½ tablespoon of oil on medium-high heat and sauté the onion for 3 to 5 minutes or until nearly translucent. Add the poblano chile and sauté for 2 to 3 minutes, or until the chile becomes bright green. Add the tomato and sauté for another 1 to 2 minutes.

3. Add the Tofu Huevos and cook for 10 minutes, stirring occasionally, to lightly brown evenly.

4. Toss in the tortillas and combine. Season with salt.

5. Serve hot with the garnishes of your choice.

ORIGIN STORY: Growing up in Brownsville—a border town on the southernmost tip of Texas—there were tortillerias (tortilla factories) on virtually every street corner. Freshly made, piping hot tortillas cost less than a quarter per dozen. My brother and I used to do tortilla runs on our bikes before dinner most evenings. The first thing we'd do was bust into one of those hot stacks, then roll up a still-steaming tortilla with our bare palms and devour it before riding back home. It's amazing we ever had leftovers, but we often did. And with those, we made migas for breakfast.

CHILAQUILES

SERVES 4 • PREP TIME: 10 MINUTES • COOK TIME: 10 MINUTES

There are many iterations of chilaquiles in contemporary Mexican cuisine. In coastal regions of Mexico, you might see them topped with fish or shrimp. In other regions, you'll find them topped with chicken or loads of cheese. This classic recipe is how we ate them at home. Like migas, chilaquiles are made with day-old corn tortillas fried in a pan or griddle until they're almost crispy. While some preparation methods include deep frying the tortilla squares, Grandma's more frugal method of pan toasting with light oil is the more traditional, cost-saving method. The goal is to get the tortillas crispy enough to give them crunch and tender enough to soak up the wonderful red salsa.

8 corn tortillas
2 tablespoons canola oil
1 cup Salsa Ranchera (page 199)
Salt

GARNISH OPTIONS
White or yellow onion, finely diced
Cilantro
Vegan shredded white cheese

1. Cut the tortillas into 1-inch squares. Heat the oil in a large pan and pan-toast the tortillas on medium-high heat, tossing the squares gently and constantly to prevent clumping.

2. When the tortilla squares are slightly crispy but still tender, add the Salsa Ranchera and heat it through. Season with salt.

3. Serve hot, topped with the garnishes of your choice.

SIMPLE SWAP: Make chilaquiles verdes (green chilaquiles) by using Roasted Tomatillo Salsa (page 201) instead of Salsa Ranchera. Garnish with Cashew Crema Mexicana (page 230) and chopped cilantro.

COOKING TIP: Want to toss this wonderful breakfast together in just 20 minutes? Use store-bought salsa in place of the Salsa Ranchera.

BORDER TOWN CORNMEAL PANQUEQUES

Nothing says comfort food like Grandma's border town panqueques—a Tex-Mex take on pancakes made with cornmeal and topped with sugared mango and banana.

FOR THE FRUIT TOPPING
2 small mangos, peeled and diced
2 bananas, peeled and sliced
⅓ cup sugar
1 tablespoon lime juice

FOR THE PANQUEQUES
¾ cup whole-wheat baking flour
½ cup cornmeal
2 teaspoons baking powder
2 tablespoons piloncillo
1 tablespoon ground cinnamon

2 tablespoons corn oil or vegetable oil
1¼ cup rice milk or other vegan milk
⅓ cup water
1 teaspoon vanilla extract
2 teaspoons grated lime zest
Nonstick cooking spray

GARNISH OPTIONS
1 tablespoon chopped fresh mint
4 to 6 tablespoons toasted
    coconut flakes

1. **TO MAKE THE FRUIT TOPPING:** In a large bowl, combine all the ingredients.

2. Mix well and set aside.

1. **TO MAKE THE PANQUEQUES:** Preheat a large nonstick skillet on medium-high heat (or heat an electric griddle on medium-high).

2. In a large bowl, combine the flour, cornmeal, baking powder, piloncillo, and cinnamon, and mix well.

3. In a separate bowl, combine the oil, rice milk, water, vanilla, and lime zest. Whisk together.

4. Fold the wet ingredients into the dry ingredients and mix with a fork until just combined. Some lumps are fine.

5. Spray the pan with nonstick cooking spray or lightly oil it. Using a ½-cup measure or ladle, pour the batter onto the pan. Cook the cakes until you see bubbles forming on top and the edges are brown, about 3 to 4 minutes. Flip the cakes and cook for another 3 to 4 minutes. Remove from the pan and keep warm. Repeat until all the batter is cooked.

6. Top the panqueques with the fruit topping and any garnishes.

SECRET INGREDIENT: Real maple syrup is also great on these cakes. Avoid the maple-flavored stuff, and insist on the real thing.

MOLLETE

SERVES 4 • PREP TIME: 10 MINUTES • COOK TIME: 15 MINUTES

Nothing gets the day going like feasting on protein-packed bean, veggie chorizo, and cheese mollete, an open-faced breakfast sandwich loaded with refried black beans, plant-based chorizo, and gooey vegan white cheese. Beans, chorizo, cheese, and bolillos are staples in most Mexican households, making mollete a popular morning meal throughout Mexico. It's also served as a starter at weekend brunch. Bolillos can be found in any Latin market and conventional grocery stores in most major US cities. If you can't find bolillos in your neck of the woods, don't sweat it. Standard French bread (cut into 6-inch slices) or plain hoagie rolls make for excellent substitutes.

4 bolillos
8 teaspoons vegan butter
1 cup Refried Black Beans (page 171)
1 to 1½ cups Garbanzorizo (page 242), or
    store-bought vegan chorizo, cooked
½ to 1 cup vegan shredded
    white cheese

GARNISH OPTIONS
1 avocado, sliced
1 to 2 cups Pico de Gallo (page 198)
1 lime, quartered

1. Preheat the oven to 350°F.

2. Cut the bolillos open. Spread 1 teaspoon of butter on the sliced side of each half. Place the bolillo halves on a baking sheet facing up and toast for 5 minutes, or until the edges are golden and crispy. Remove from the oven.

3. Spread 2 tablespoons of Refried Black Beans evenly over each bread half. Top the beans with 2 to 3 tablespoons of Garbanzorizo or chorizo. Sprinkle 1 to 2 tablespoons of the shredded cheese over each half and place back in oven for 5 minutes, or until the cheese has melted.

4. Serve with the garnishes of your choice.

COOKING TIP: For a sweet mollete, spread butter on the bread and sprinkle each half with 1 teaspoon of sugar. Toast for 5 to 7 minutes or until the edges are golden brown. Sprinkle with cinnamon and serve.

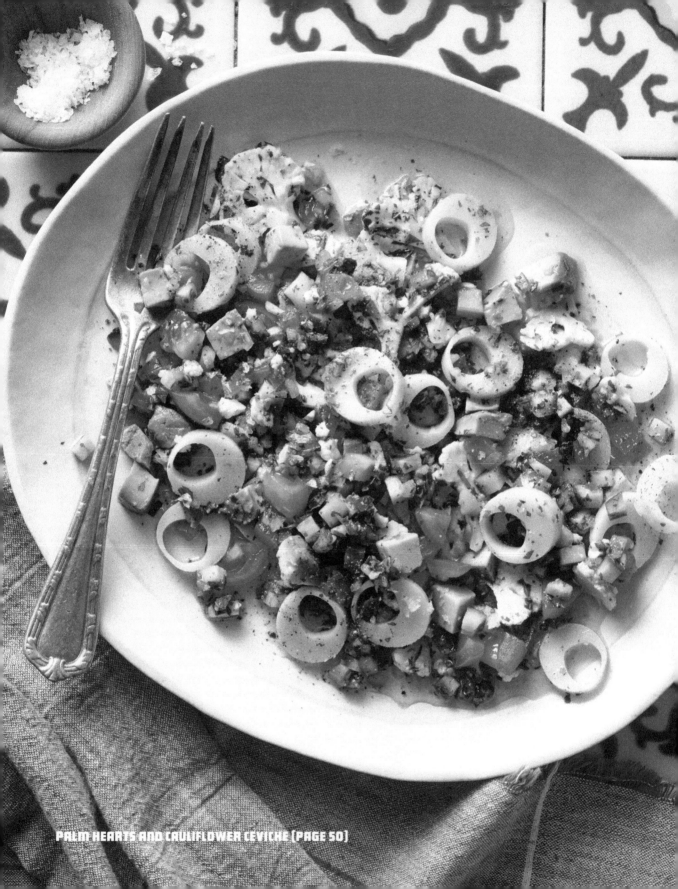

PALM HEARTS AND CAULIFLOWER CEVICHE (PAGE 50)

Chapter 3

SALADS, SOUPS, AND STEWS

SPICY WATERMELON AND JICAMA SALAD

SERVES 4 • PREP TIME: 15 MINUTES

Imagine it's August. The sun is beating down. You're sitting out by the pool, or maybe just relaxing in the park with a few friends and a picnic. There's nothing better than biting into a sweet, juicy watermelon on that hot summer day. And this recipe for spicy watermelon salad is perfect for bringing a little bit of that summer heat into every bite. This sweet and savory fruit salad features watermelon, jicama, julienned jalapeño, cilantro, and lime for a delicious, balanced blend of sweet and heat.

1 small seedless watermelon (about 1½ pounds), skinned and diced medium
1 small jicama (about ¾ pounds), peeled and julienned
1 jalapeño chile, seeded and julienned

Zest of 2 limes
Juice of 4 limes
¼ teaspoon salt
¼ cup toasted unsweetened coconut
¼ cup chopped cilantro

1. In a large bowl, mix together the watermelon, jicama, jalapeño, and lime zest.

2. Add the lime juice and salt and toss gently.

3. Top with the coconut and cilantro.

SECRET INGREDIENT: Look for a watermelon that's heavy for its size, and knock on its underside to listen for a hollow sound. This will ensure your watermelon is perfectly juicy and ripe.

FRUTERIA-STYLE FRUIT SALAD

SERVES 4 TO 6 • PREP TIME: 20 MINUTES

Originally from the Chiapas and Veracruz regions of southern Mexico, papaya is now a staple throughout Latin America. Combined with mango and jicama—and topped with shredded coconut, chili powder, and cinnamon—this fruit salad has always been a family favorite at Garza gatherings. The goal here is to let the sweetness of the mango and papaya combine with the mild flavor of the jicama, and just tickle the taste buds with a hint of chili and cinnamon.

1 papaya, peeled, seeded, and
   diced medium
1 jicama, peeled and diced medium
2 mangos, peeled and diced medium
Juice of 1 lime
Salt
1 teaspoon chili powder

1 teaspoon ground cinnamon
¼ teaspoon cayenne pepper
2 tablespoons Aztec Spiced
   Pepitas (page 69)
2 tablespoons unsweetened
   coconut shreds

1. Place the papaya, jicama, and mangos in a large mixing bowl.

2. Add the lime juice and salt and toss gently.

3. Top with the chili powder, cinnamon, cayenne, Aztec Spiced Pepitas, and coconut shreds.

SECRET INGREDIENT: To find the perfect papaya, look for a fruit that is mostly yellow or orange (a few green spots are fine). Press the papaya gently with your fingertips; they should sink slightly into the fruit when it's ready to eat, just like an avocado.

CHIRIMOYA-JICAMA SALAD

SERVES 6 • PREP TIME: 15 MINUTES, PLUS 30 MINUTES CHILLING TIME

Mark Twain called the chirimoya "the most delicious fruit known to man." This easy-to-make chirimoya-jicama salad is the perfect fruit combo for any summer occasion. Whether you're headed to the beach, a lakeside picnic, or a summer piñata party, guests will love this tropical combination of creamy chirimoya, crisp jicama, and juicy pineapple and mango. Sweet potato (yes, raw) and olive oil offer a warm balance to this otherwise bright fruit blend, and the dash of salt really brings out the fruits' robust flavors.

Juice of 1 lemon
½ cup olive oil
1 teaspoon balsamic vinegar
Pinch of salt
1 mango, peeled, seeded, and sliced into thin strips
2 cups chopped pineapple

2 ripe chirimoyas, peeled, seeded, and cut into cubes
1 large jicama, peeled and sliced into thin strips
1 medium sweet potato, peeled and grated

1. In a small bowl, whisk together the lemon juice, oil, vinegar, and salt.

2. In a large bowl, and toss the mango, pineapple, chirimoyas, jicama, and sweet potato.

3. Pour on the dressing and toss gently to combine.

4. Chill 30 to 45 minutes before serving.

SECRET INGREDIENT: A chirimoya is ripe when the skin is mostly brown. Many Latin markets and most Asian markets carry them. Can't find chirimoyas in your neck of the woods? No problem. Simply replace it with half a banana (diced) and one peach (peeled and diced).

GRILLED NOPAL SALAD

SF

GF

SERVES 4 • PREP TIME: 20 MINUTES • COOK TIME: 10 MINUTES

Grilled nopal cactus pads—sometimes called "green steaks"—make the perfect topping for this delicious summer salad. Like grilled asparagus, they have a bright, robust flavor. At my childhood home, we grew nopales in our backyard and my favorite way to eat them was grilled to a char but still al dente. This green salad, topped with avocado, perfectly grilled nopales, and Cashew Crema Mexicana dressing (the recipe yields 2 cups), will have you firing up the grill all summer!

FOR THE DRESSING

1 avocado, peeled, seeded, and roughly chopped

5 tablespoons Cashew Crema Mexicana (page 230)

Juice of 3 limes

2 tablespoons apple cider vinegar

½ jalapeño chile, or more if you like it hot

Salt

Freshly ground black pepper

¼ to ½ cup water

¼ bunch cilantro, roughly chopped

FOR THE SALAD

3 nopal cactus pads, dethorned and peeled

2 tablespoons olive oil

Juice of 1 lime

Salt

Freshly ground black pepper

1 head green leaf, red leaf, or romaine lettuce, cut into bite-size pieces

2 to 3 cups baby spinach, arugula, or a mix of spring greens

1 carrot, peeled and julienned

½ medium red onion, julienned

1 red bell pepper, seeded and julienned

10 radishes, thinly sliced, divided

1 Roma tomato, seeded and julienned

½ cucumber, peeled, sliced on an angle

½ cup Aztec Spiced Roasted Hominy (page 71)

⅓ cup Almond Queso Cotija (page 73)

1. TO MAKE THE DRESSING: In a blender, purée until smooth the avocado, Cashew Crema Mexicana, lime juice, apple cider vinegar, jalapeño, salt, and pepper, along with just enough water to get the blender moving. Add more water as needed to get a nice dressing consistency.

2. Add the cilantro and blend about 1 minute more. Set aside.

1. TO MAKE THE SALAD: Preheat the grill to medium-high heat.

2. Toss the prepared cactus with olive oil and lime juice. Season with salt and pepper. Grill for 5 to 7 minutes on each side. You want a nice char and the cactus to be al dente. Remove from the heat. Let them cool until you can handle the cactus. Cut into bite-size strips.

3. If you don't have a grill, in a hot cast-iron skillet, sear the nopales on medium-high heat for about 5 minutes on each side.

4. In a large bowl, toss the lettuce, greens, carrot, onion, bell pepper, and 6 radishes. Dress with 2 to 4 tablespoons of dressing. (You'll have plenty of extra dressing to use later, which you can store in the refrigerator for up to 5 days.) Transfer to a serving bowl. Top with the tomatos, cucumber, the remaining radishes, and warm cactus.

5. Sprinkle with Aztec Spiced Roasted Hominy and Almond Queso Cotija.

SECRET INGREDIENT: Nopales can be found at most Latin markets already de-thorned and peeled. If you're cleaning them yourself, hold the pad on a slant and scrape downward with a sharp knife toward the tip of the pad to remove the thorns. Cut off any remaining thorns one at a time.

PALM HEARTS 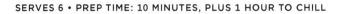 CAULIFLOWER CEVICHE

SERVES 6 • PREP TIME: 10 MINUTES, PLUS 1 HOUR TO CHILL

Ceviche, a dish known for its refreshing flavors and unique textures, now comes to you in an entirely plant-based form, thanks to hearts of palm and cauliflower. Various kinds of seafood have found their way into different ceviches over the years, but for this recipe, I go for multilayered hearts of palm. Hearts of palm can mimic both scallops and calamari rings when the center of the palm heart is separated from its outer ring. By chopping raw cauliflower into small pieces, we are able to pack a soft crunch into the dish, ensuring that this new ceviche delivers on both texture and freshness.

2 large Roma tomatoes, diced
    into cubes
1 cup chopped red onion
1 cup chopped cilantro
2 jalapeño chiles, seeded
    and chopped
1 cucumber, diced into cubes
1 cup finely chopped cauliflower

1 (14-ounce) can hearts of palm,
    drained, centers pushed out, cut
    into slices
1 tablespoon olive oil
Juice of 2 lemons
1 avocado, peeled, seeded, and diced
Salt
Freshly ground black pepper

1. In a large bowl, combine the tomatoes, onion, cilantro, jalapeños, cucumber, and cauliflower. Mix well.

2. Add the hearts of palm, olive oil, and lemon juice, and mix.

3. Add the avocado, season with salt and pepper, and toss gently.

4. Chill for at least 1 hour before serving.

COOKING TIP: This hearty ceviche recipe is served best on its own, or with saltine crackers.

AZTEC SEARED CHICKEN-STYLE SETAS SALAD

SF

GF

SERVES 4 • PREP TIME: 15 MINUTES • COOK TIME: 15 TO 20 MINUTES

On their own, setas (oyster mushrooms) offer the perfect mild taste and soft texture to mimic chicken and other types of meat. These functional fungi—found in tropical climates across the world—are robust and hearty, and this spicy rub and flavorful preparation will really bring out their meaty qualities. The chili-lime vinaigrette offers a bit of tartness and heat, while the roasted pumpkin seeds pack a protein punch.

FOR THE CHILI LIME VINAIGRETTE
⅓ cup olive oil
4 tablespoons apple cider vinegar
2 tablespoons lime juice
1 teaspoon dark chili powder
¼ teaspoon salt
¼ teaspoon freshly ground
    black pepper
1 tablespoon chopped cilantro

FOR THE SALAD
1 recipe Seared Chicken-Style Setas
    (page 238)
½ cup frozen or fresh corn kernels
12 cherry or grape tomatoes
One head red leaf lettuce or romaine,
    roughly chopped
2 cups bitter greens, such as frisée or
    arugula, separated
½ medium red onion, julienned
4 to 5 radishes, sliced into thin wheels
Freshly ground black pepper
Chopped cilantro
2 tablespoons Aztec Spiced Pepitas
    (page 69)

1. TO MAKE THE CHILI LIME VINAIGRETTE:
In a small bowl, whisk together the oil, vinegar, and lime juice.

2. Add the chili powder, salt, pepper, and cilantro, and whisk for about 1 more minute. The oil and vinegar should not be fully emulsified.

3. Set aside.

1. TO MAKE THE SALAD: Prepare the Seared Chicken-Style Setas.

2. Use the same cast-iron skillet as the setas to sauté the corn for 4 to 5 minutes, or until it is nicely caramelized. Set the corn aside. Add the tomatoes, whole, and cook until they pop and blister, about 5 minutes. Remove from the heat.

Continued

3. To assemble the salad, in a large bowl toss the lettuce and greens, onion, and radishes with a small amount of dressing. Transfer to a large dinner plate. Top with the Seared Chicken-Style Setas, corn, and blistered tomatoes.

4. Add the pepper, chopped cilantro, and Aztec Spiced Pepitas. Serve with extra dressing on the side.

SIMPLE SWAP: I like using oyster mushrooms for most recipes that call for chicken. But if mushrooms aren't your thing, simply toss your favorite brand of chicken-free strips with my Aztec Spice Blend (page 229) and sear as in the Seared Chicken-Style Setas recipe.

MEXICAN-STYLE GAZPACHO

SERVES 4 • PREP TIME: 15 MINUTES, PLUS 1 HOUR CHILLING TIME •
COOK TIME: 15 MINUTES

Gazpacho is a chilled tomato, cucumber, and garlic soup that originated in the southern Spanish region of Andalusia. There are now variations of gazpacho in virtually all Hispanic cuisines, featuring an assortment of locally available ingredients. Grandma's Mexican gazpacho always included fresh corn, shaved directly off the cob, and jalapeños. Garnished with avocado, cilantro, radish relish, and then drizzled with cashew cream, this chilled soup is a delightful starter to any summertime meal.

4 large ripe Roma tomatoes, quartered
1 medium cucumber, peeled and
   roughly chopped
1 large jalapeño chile, seeded
   and quartered
1 shallot, peeled and quartered
1 to 2 garlic cloves, quartered
2 tablespoons apple cider vinegar
½ teaspoon dried Mexican oregano
½ teaspoon salt
Freshly ground black pepper
¼ cup olive oil

GARNISH OPTIONS
¼ cup fresh cilantro or parsley,
   chopped
Kernels from 1 ear of fresh corn
1 avocado, peeled, seeded, and diced
½ cup Cashew Crema Mexicana
   (page 230)
½ cup Red Onion, Radish, and Cilantro
   Relish (page 205)

1. In a blender or food processor, process the tomatoes into a rough purée. Add the cucumber, jalapeño, shallot, garlic, vinegar, oregano, salt, and pepper, and blend until mostly smooth.

2. With the blender or processor still running, slowly pour in the olive oil and blend until the soup is smooth and all the ingredients are well integrated.

3. Pour the soup in a large container and cover. Chill for at least 1 hour before serving.

4. Serve the soup cold with the garnishes of your choice.

SIMPLE SWAP: To make this soup nut-free, simply omit the Cashew Crema Mexicana.

MEXICAN LENTIL SOUP

SF

GF

NF

SERVES 8 • PREP TIME: 10 MINUTES • COOK TIME: 60 MINUTES

Lentils pack in more protein than virtually any other legume. They date back to Neolithic times, and today are used to prepare healthy and affordable dishes across the world. This lentil-laden soup is enjoyed throughout Mexico and Central America, and features rich vegetable stock, stewed tomatoes, celery, cumin, and other flavorful ingredients that will fill any home with mouthwatering aromas and any hungry stomach with nourishment.

1 tablespoon olive oil
1 large carrot, peeled and diced small
1 medium onion, diced
3 celery stalks, diced small
3 garlic cloves, minced
1 tablespoon ground cumin
1 teaspoon dried Mexican oregano
1 teaspoon salt
1 teaspoon freshly ground black pepper
2 chipotles in adobo, minced, plus
    2 tablespoons adobo sauce from
    the can

3 cups lentils
1 large russet potato, peeled and
    diced small
1 (15-ounce) can diced tomatoes,
    not drained
10 cups Homemade Vegetable Stock
    (page 231)
3 tablespoons minced cilantro
2 limes, quartered

1. Heat a large soup pot over medium-high heat. Add the oil and sauté the carrot, onion, celery, and garlic for 5 to 7 minutes.

2. Add the cumin, oregano, salt, and pepper, and stir. Then add the chipotle chiles and sauté for 2 minutes. Add the adobo sauce, lentils, potato, tomatoes and their juice, Homemade Vegetable Stock, and cilantro, and bring to a boil.

3. Reduce the heat to a simmer and cook, covered, for 40 to 50 minutes. The lentils should remain intact and still have their shape, but be cooked through.

4. Serve hot with a lime wedge.

COOKING TIP: If you overcook the lentils, have no fear. Just pulse them with an immersion blender or in a regular blender and enjoy as a smooth puréed soup. Adding some steamed rice can help make this bowl even more satisfying.

TORTILLA SOUP

SERVES 8 • PREP TIME: 15 MINUTES • COOK TIME: 50 MINUTES

The origins of tortilla soup are largely unknown. Some sources say it originated in Central Mexico; others argue it originated in the American Southwest in the 1960s. What I can tell you for sure is that it's absolutely delicious and remains a Garza family favorite! My tortilla soup features soy crumbles in place of the chicken Grandma used in her recipe. Feel free to swap soy crumbles for any of the chicken alternatives on the market.

2 dried pasilla chiles
2 dried ancho chiles
2 tablespoons tomato paste
2 (15-ounce) cans diced tomatoes, not drained
1 tablespoon olive oil
1 carrot, peeled and diced medium
1 medium onion, diced medium
2 celery stalks, diced medium
5 garlic cloves, minced
2 cups TVP, rehydrated 15 minutes in 1½ cups water
2 teaspoons ground cumin
2 teaspoons dried Mexican oregano
1 teaspoon salt
2 teaspoons freshly ground black pepper

8 cups Homemade Vegetable Stock (page 231)
1 (15-ounce) can black beans, drained and rinsed
2 cups frozen corn kernels, thawed
¼ cup chopped cilantro or fresh epazote
Juice of 2 limes

GARNISH OPTIONS
2 avocados, peeled, seeded, and diced
Broken tortilla chips, or pan fried tortilla strips
3 limes, quartered
4 radishes, julienned
½ bunch cilantro, chopped
1 cup vegan shredded white cheese

1. Toast the pasilla and ancho chiles in a dry pan over medium heat, about 7 minutes on each side. They are ready when your kitchen smells great from the toasted chiles. Then remove the seeds and stems and rip the chiles into pieces.

2. In a blender, blend the chiles, tomato paste, tomatoes, and their juice on high for about 2 to 3 minutes.

3. In a large soup pot on medium heat, add the oil and sauté the carrot, onion, celery, and garlic for about 7 to 10 minutes, or until soft.

4. Add them to the blender with the tomatoes and blend until smooth.

5. In the same pot on medium heat, sauté the rehydrated TVP and the cumin, oregano, salt, and pepper for

Continued

about 4 minutes. Pour in the tomato mixture from the blender and simmer for 5 minutes.

6. Add the Homemade Vegetable Stock and bring to a boil. Reduce the heat to a simmer and cook, uncovered, for 15 minutes.

7. Add in the beans, corn, cilantro or epazote, and lime juice, and cook 5 minutes more.

8. Serve in bowls with the garnishes of your choice.

HEAT INDEX: This recipe has a heat level of 6 out of 10. Increase the heat by adding in 1 to 2 chipotles or 2 teaspoons of red chili flakes to the blender in step 2.

SOPA DE FIDEO

SERVES 4 • PREP TIME: 10 MINUTES • COOK TIME: 20 MINUTES

Sopa de Fideo (pronounced fee-DAY-oh*) is a traditional noodle soup popular throughout Mexico and the Southwestern US. It's prepared with distinctive spices and special additions in different regions, but the cooking method is what characterizes this wonderful noodle soup. All Sopas de Fideo start by toasting the noodles, giving them a rich nutty flavor, and simmering them in a tomato-based sauce. The soup can serve as a main dish by adding seitan crumbles or any other hearty plant-based protein, or it can be a delicious starter or side dish.*

1 tablespoon olive oil
1 (7-ounce) package dry fideo noodles
3 cups Homemade Vegetable Stock
   (page 231)
1 teaspoon ground cumin
¼ teaspoon chipotle powder
1 teaspoon salt

4 medium Roma tomatoes, quartered
2 garlic cloves
½ large yellow onion, quartered
2 cups water
½ cup chopped cilantro
1 lime, quartered

1. In a large stockpot, heat the oil and sauté the noodles until golden brown, stirring frequently and being careful not to burn them. Add the Homemade Vegetable Stock, cumin, chipotle powder, and salt, and reduce the heat to a simmer.

2. In a blender, combine the tomatoes, garlic, onion, and water and purée until smooth. Add the purée to the soup pot, and cook over medium-low heat for 15 to 20 minutes.

3. Serve hot, garnished with cilantro and a lime wedge.

SECRET INGREDIENT: Fideo is a thin, very short noodle. If you can't find it, substitute vermicelli or angel hair pasta, broken into pieces.

COOKING TIP: This recipe comes together in just 20 minutes if you have ready-made vegetable stock.

SEVEN SEAS SOUP

SERVES 8 • PREP TIME: 30 MINUTES, PLUS 40 TO 60 MINUTES SOAKING TIME • COOK TIME: 1 HOUR

I grew up eating this Mexican seafood stew and, after becoming vegan, always pined for a fish-free version. This recipe features a rich tomato and dulse broth and features hearty potatoes, delicious palm and artichoke hearts, and protein-packed chickpeas. Each time I cook it, I'm immediately transported back to my childhood home and Grandma's cooking.

8 dried guajillo chiles
2 tablespoons vegetable oil, divided
4 garlic cloves, minced
½ tablespoon dried Mexican oregano
1 teaspoon salt
½ teaspoon freshly ground black pepper
2 teaspoons ground cumin
2 teaspoons dark chili powder
1 teaspoon smoked paprika
1 to 2 tablespoons dulse flakes
1 (15.5-ounce) can whole tomatoes, not drained
1 (8-ounce) can tomato sauce
2 carrots, diced medium
1 medium onion, diced medium

3 celery stalks, diced medium
1 large russet potato, diced medium
4 cups Homemade Vegetable Stock (page 231)
1 (14-ounce) can hearts of palm, drained, roughly chopped, keeping some of the round rings whole
1 (13.75-ounce) can artichoke hearts, drained and roughly chopped
3 ears fresh corn on the cob, cut into quarters
2 calabacita squashes, diced medium
1 (15.5-ounce) can chickpeas, not drained
½ bunch cilantro, chopped
Lime wedges, for garnish

1. Soak the guajillo chiles in hot water for 1 hour (or microwave for 10 minutes and let sit for 30 minutes, covered). Then seed and chop them.

2. Heat 1 tablespoon of oil in a large soup pot, and sauté the garlic, oregano, salt, pepper, cumin, chili powder, paprika, and dulse flakes for 3 minutes, bringing together into a paste. Add the rehydrated chiles, tomatoes and their juice, and tomato sauce. Lower the heat and simmer for 10 minutes.

3. Purée the soup base in a blender (in batches), or blend with an immersion blender and remove it from the pot. Set aside.

4. In the same pot, heat 1 tablespoon of oil on medium heat and sauté the carrots, onion, and celery for 3 minutes.

Return the soup base to the pot. Add the potato and Homemade Vegetable Stock, and cook for 10 to 15 minutes or until the potato is tender.

5. Add the hearts of palm, artichoke hearts, corn on the cob, calabacitas, and chickpeas with their aquafaba liquid. Cook for 5 to 7 minutes.

6. Serve hot, garnished with cilantro and lime wedges.

SECRET INGREDIENT: Calabacitas can be found at any Latin market. They look like a cross between zucchini and yellow summer squash. If you can't find calabacitas, use either zucchini or summer squash.

AZTEC SPICED PUMPKIN SOUP

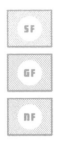

SERVES 8 • PREP TIME: 20 MINUTES • COOK TIME: 90 MINUTES

As a kid I would wait eagerly for pumpkin season, when I could enjoy the orange squash in all its forms. This soup features puréed aromatic pumpkin drizzled with a rich cashew cream that blends wonderfully into the spiced soup. The crunchy roasted pumpkin seeds on top add a perfect pop.

3 tablespoons olive oil
1 tablespoon Aztec Spice Blend (page 229)
2 teaspoons salt
1 teaspoon freshly ground black pepper
3 tablespoons Classic Chile Paste (page 194)
1 medium pumpkin, quartered and seeded, skin on
1 large onion, diced
2 carrots, peeled and diced medium
3 celery stalks, diced medium

6 garlic cloves, smashed and roughly chopped
2 serrano chiles, seeded and diced small
2 large russet potatoes, peeled and diced medium
12 cups Homemade Vegetable Stock (page 231)

GARNISH OPTIONS
Cashew Crema Mexicana (page 230)
Aztec Spiced Pepitas (page 69)

1. Preheat the oven to 350°F.

2. Mix the oil, Aztec Spice Blend, salt, pepper, and Classic Chile Paste in a small bowl. Rub the flesh side of the pumpkin with the mixture, saving about 1 tablespoon for the remaining vegetables.

3. In a large roasting pan, roast the pumpkin for 40 minutes.

4. Toss the onion, carrots, celery, garlic, and serrano chiles in the remaining 1 tablespoon of seasoning mix and add to the pan with the pumpkin. Roast 20 minutes more. When all the vegetables are cooked, scoop out the roasted pumpkin and discard the skin.

5. Heat a large soup pot on medium-high heat and toss in all the roasted vegetables and the potatoes. Pour in the Homemade Vegetable Stock and bring to a boil. Reduce the heat and simmer, covered, for 20 minutes.

6. Using an immersion blender (or a regular blender, in batches), purée the soup until smooth. If the soup is too thick, add more vegetable stock to bring it to a nice consistency.

7. Top with the garnishes of your choice, and serve hot.

SIMPLE SWAP: If you would like to garnish the soup with a cream topping while keeping the soup nut-free, try a dollop of soy-based sour cream. Tofutti brand is completely nut-free and manufactured in nut-free facilities.

SEAFOOD-STYLE POZOLE

SERVES 6 TO 8 • PREP TIME: 10 MINUTES • COOK TIME: 30 MINUTES

Pozole means "hominy," a traditional Central American food made from large dried maize kernels that features prominently in this classic Mexican stew. Seafood pozole is typically found in coastal regions of Mexico and is served at celebrations like quinceañeras and birthdays, and for the New Year. Today, it's a popular menu item at Mexican restaurants all over the world. Pozole in coastal regions of Mexico traditionally contains fish or other sea animals. This version features soft, elegant hearts of palm instead.

1 tablespoon olive oil
1 medium onion, diced small
6 garlic cloves, minced
2 to 3 tablespoons Classic Chile Paste (page 194)
½ tablespoon ground cumin
1 (15-ounce) can hearts of palm, drained and sliced in rings
1 tablespoon dulse flakes
1 teaspoon salt
1 teaspoon freshly ground black pepper

2 (15-ounce) cans hominy, drained and rinsed
1 (15-ounce) can diced tomatoes, not drained
12 cups Homemade Vegetable Stock (page 231)

GARNISH OPTIONS
Sliced radishes
Chopped cilantro
Chopped raw onions

1. In a large soup pot, heat the oil on medium-high heat and sauté the onion and garlic for 5 minutes. Add the Classic Chile Paste and cumin and sauté for 3 more minutes.

2. Add the hearts of palm and sauté for about 2 minutes, stirring gently so as not to break all the rings.

3. Add the dulse, salt, pepper, hominy, tomatoes and their juice, and Homemade Vegetable Stock. Bring to a boil, then simmer, uncovered, for 20 minutes.

4. Serve hot with the garnishes of your choice.

SIMPLE SWAP: This pozole is based on a seafood dish we typically made at home in my coastal hometown of Brownsville, Texas. Try using your favorite brand of plant-based chicken in place of the palm hearts, and omit the dulse flakes for a different variation.

GUISO DE FLOR DE CALABAZA

MAKES 4 • PREP TIME: 10 MINUTES • COOK TIME: 20 MINUTES

Squash blossoms are not only beautiful, but their complex flavor will leave guests in awe. You can find them when summer squash and zucchini are in season, as well as on late harvest pumpkins. Squash blossoms are light and have a hint of citrus. In Mexico, these delicate edible flowers are used in all sorts of dishes, including quesadillas, soups, and salads. In this recipe, the blossoms accompany ripe Roma tomatoes, jalapeño, and onion for a healthy and satisfying guiso—a quick stew.

1 tablespoon vegetable oil
1 medium red onion, julienned
1 large jalapeño chile, seeded and julienned
2 garlic cloves, minced
2 Roma tomatoes, seeded and julienned

10 fresh zucchini blossoms, roughly chopped
½ teaspoon fresh lime juice
2 tablespoons chopped cilantro
½ teaspoon salt
¼ teaspoon freshly ground black pepper

1. In a large skillet, heat the oil on medium-high heat. Sauté the onion and jalapeño for 7 minutes.

2. Add the garlic, tomatoes, and blossoms, and sauté for 5 minutes more. Turn off the heat.

3. Stir in the lime and cilantro. Season with salt and pepper.

SECRET INGREDIENT: When picking squash blossoms from your own vegetable garden, make sure you pick the fuzzier ones with a thin base at the stem. Those are the male blossoms. Female blossoms, which have a thick bulge near the flower, are what actually become the fruit.

PICADILLO

SERVES 6 • PREP TIME: 10 MINUTES • COOK TIME: 30 MINUTES

Picadillo is a classic stew enjoyed throughout northern Mexico. Tomato-based and packed with meat-free beef crumbles and potatoes, this dish is as robust as any meat-based stew. Served on its own, over a bed of rice, or in a savory empanada, this picadillo will satisfy and delight even the most ardent meat eater.

1 tablespoon vegetable oil
1 medium onion, diced small
3 garlic cloves, minced
1 or 2 serrano chiles, seeded and
    diced small
½ tablespoon whole cumin seeds
2 cups TVP, rehydrated with 1½ cups
    hot water, crumbled
2 medium russet potatoes, peeled
    and diced medium

1 (15-ounce) can diced tomatoes,
    not drained
4 cups Homemade Vegetable
    Stock (page 231)
¼ tablespoon apple cider vinegar
½ teaspoon salt
½ teaspoon freshly ground
    black pepper
3 tablespoons chopped cilantro

1. Heat a large soup pot on medium-high heat. Add the oil and sauté the onion, garlic, serrano chiles, and cumin seeds for 3 to 5 minutes. Add the rehydrated TVP crumbles and potatoes and sauté for 3 to 5 more minutes.

2. Add the tomatoes and their juice, Homemade Vegetable Stock, vinegar, salt, and pepper, and bring to boil. Reduce the heat to a simmer and cook, uncovered, for 20 minutes.

3. Stir in the cilantro and serve hot.

SECRET INGREDIENT: This recipe calls for TVP because it's widely available in Mexico and sold in bulk in the produce section of many Latin markets across the US. Feel free to substitute your favorite brand of beefy crumbles.

RED CHILI SEITAN STEAK AND BEAN GUISADO

SERVES 4 • PREP TIME: 15 MINUTES • COOK TIME: 20 MINUTES

Guisados, or stews, offer a burst of heartiness and flavor, and are essential in Mexican and other Latin American cuisines. Here we bring a healthy and modern update to a northern Mexican ranch-style classic by pairing seitan "steak" with a red sauce and beans. Imagine cooking over a campfire under a clear northern Mexican evening sky.

2 tablespoons vegetable oil

1 white onion, diced medium

2 chipotle chiles in adobo sauce, minced, plus 2 tablespoons adobo sauce from the can

1 green bell pepper, seeded and diced medium

3 garlic cloves, minced

2 tablespoons chili powder

½ teaspoon whole cumin seeds

¼ teaspoon dried Mexican oregano

½ teaspoon salt

½ teaspoon freshly ground black pepper

1 pound Mexican Seasoned Seitan (page 239), diced medium

1 (15-ounce) can diced tomatoes, not drained

1 cup Homemade Vegetable Stock (page 231), divided

½ cup dark Mexican lager

1 tablespoon cornstarch

1 (15-ounce) can black beans, drained and rinsed

1. Heat the oil in a large skillet over high heat. Sauté the onion, chipotle, and bell pepper for 5 minutes. Add the garlic, chili powder, cumin, oregano, salt, pepper, and Mexican Seasoned Seitan. Cook until the seitan is well-browned, about 5 minutes.

2. Add the tomatoes and their juice, and all but 2 tablespoons of Homemade Vegetable Stock (save that 2 tablespoons to mix with the cornstarch). Add the adobo sauce from the chipotles and the lager, and bring to a boil.

3. Reduce the heat to a simmer. Cook, uncovered, for 10 minutes.

4. In a small bowl or measuring cup, mix together the cornstarch and remaining 2 tablespoons of cold Homemade Vegetable Stock until smooth. Whisk the slurry into the skillet with the guisado. When the mixture returns to a simmer, it is thick enough.

5. Add the beans and heat through, approximately 3 to 4 minutes.

6. Serve over your favorite rice or use to fill a bread or tortilla.

HEAT INDEX: In terms of spiciness, this guisado is a 6 out of 10. For true Norteño heat, add 1 teaspoon of Chiles de Árbol Salsa (page 203) in step 5.

CHILI SIN CARNE

SERVES 6 • PREP TIME: 10 MINUTES • COOK TIME: 30 MINUTES

The name of this dish comes from the Aztec word chili, *of course referring to a chile pepper. Combined with tomatoes, garlic, onion, beans, and other ingredients, chili as a dish dates back to the mid-19th century. It was first popularized at the Chicago World's Fair, when the San Antonio Chili Stand dished up the delicious stew to fairgoers. This chili, featuring spicy beans and soy beef crumbles, is a meat-free take on the classic dish.*

1 tablespoon vegetable oil
1 onion, diced medium
1 jalapeño chile, seeded and diced
1 serrano chile, seeded and diced
4 garlic cloves, minced
2 tablespoons ground cumin
1 teaspoon salt
1 teaspoon freshly ground black pepper
3 tablespoons Classic Chile Paste
    (page 194)
2 cups TVP, rehydrated with 1½ cups
    hot water, crumbled

1 (15-ounce) can diced tomatoes,
    not drained
1 (15-ounce) can tomato sauce
1 (15-ounce) can pinto beans,
    not drained
2 cups Homemade Vegetable Stock
    (page 231)
2 teaspoons apple cider vinegar

GARNISH OPTIONS
Lime wedges
Chopped cilantro
Raw onions, diced small

1. Heat a large soup pot on medium-high heat. Add the oil and sauté the onion, jalapeño and serrano chiles, and garlic for 5 minutes, or until they are caramelized. Add the cumin, salt, pepper, and Classic Chile Paste, and cook for 2 more minutes.

2. Add the rehydrated TVP and combine. Sauté for 2 more minutes.

3. Add the tomatoes and their juice, tomato sauce, beans and aquafaba (bean liquid), Homemade Vegetable Stock, and vinegar, and reduce the heat to a simmer. Cook for 15 to 20 minutes.

4. Top with the garnishes of your choice.

HEAT INDEX: This chili is similar in taste to Wolf brand chili, my brother Michael's favorite canned brand growing up. To add more depth and heat, simply add 1 teaspoon of chipotle powder along with the chile paste.

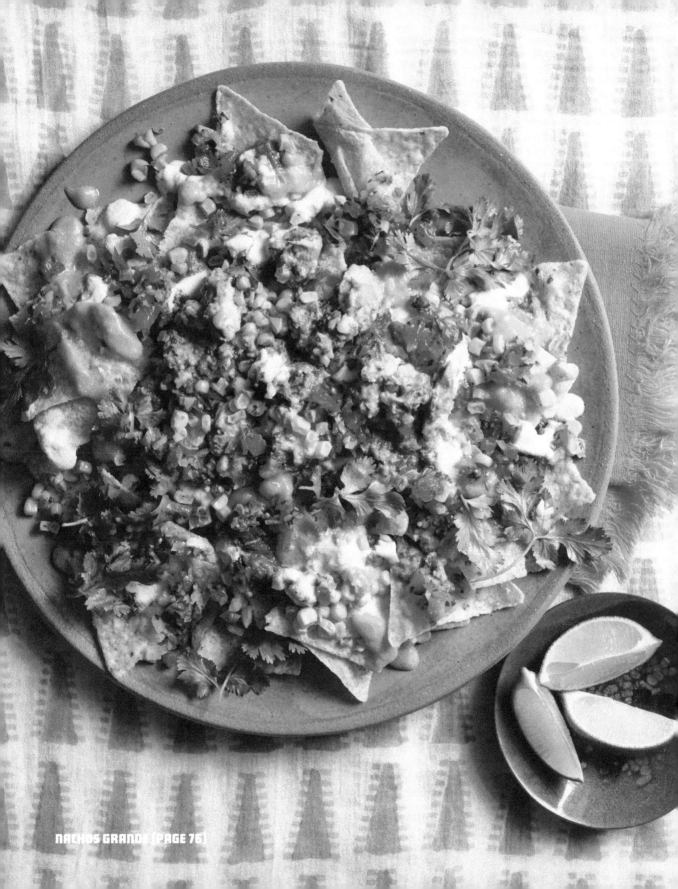

NACHOS GRANDE (PAGE 76)

Chapter 4

SNACKS AND APPETIZERS

AZTEC SPICED PEPITAS

SERVES 8 • PREP TIME: 5 MINUTES • COOK TIME: 6 TO 10 MINUTES

Pumpkin pies and sugar and spice are certainly nice, but one of the best Mexican fall flavors is roasted pumpkin seeds. They also pack a protein punch, providing more than 8 grams of protein per serving. Also called "pepitas," pumpkin seeds have a deliciously nutty flavor that is only intensified by roasting. Roasted with my signature Aztec Spice Blend, there's even more reason to have a stash of these nutritional powerhouses on hand.

1 pound raw, unsalted, shelled pumpkin seeds
1 to 2 tablespoons Aztec Spice Blend (page 229)

1 tablespoon peanut oil or other vegetable oil
¼ teaspoon salt
Juice of 1 lime

1. Preheat the oven to 350°F. Line a baking sheet with parchment paper.

2. Toss all the ingredients in a large bowl, mixing well to coat the pumpkin seeds.

3. Evenly spread the coated pumpkin seeds on the baking sheet. Roast for 5 to 7 minutes.

4. Stir the seeds and roast another 1 to 3 minutes. The pumpkin seeds should be nicely roasted and aromatic, but not burned. Watch them carefully.

COOKING TIP: You can also pan toast these on the stovetop. Heat a large skillet over medium heat and add the coated pumpkin seeds. Stir constantly with a wooden spoon for about 5 to 7 minutes.

CHILI ROASTED PEANUTS

SERVES 8 • PREP TIME: 5 MINUTES • COOK TIME: 6 TO 10 MINUTES

Chili-roasted peanuts could be considered the ultimate snack food. Not only are they quick and easy to make, but they're also packed with protein and can be made way ahead of time for any occasion. Peanuts have been cultivated in Mexico since Mesoamerican times. These spicy roasted peanuts are the perfect Aztec-inspired snack food to enjoy on movie nights or road trips, or as table munchies for quinceañeras, birthdays, and weddings. Or add them to your favorite trail mix to make a nice spicy blend.

1 pound raw, unsalted, shelled peanuts
1 tablespoon dark chili powder
½ teaspoon chipotle powder
½ teaspoon sweet paprika

1 tablespoon peanut oil or other vegetable oil
¼ teaspoon salt
Juice of 1 lime

1. Preheat the oven to 350°F. Line a baking sheet with parchment paper.

2. Toss all the ingredients in a large bowl, mixing well to coat the peanuts.

3. Evenly spread the coated peanuts on the baking sheet. Roast for 5 to 7 minutes.

4. Stir the peanuts and roast another 1 to 3 minutes. The peanuts should be nicely roasted and aromatic, but not burned. Watch them carefully.

HEAT INDEX: Feel free to tweak the amount of chili and chipotle powders based on your own heat preferences. I like to kick up the heat by adding an extra teaspoon of chipotle powder.

AZTEC SPICED ROASTED HOMINY

SERVES 8 • PREP TIME: 5 MINUTES • COOK TIME: 15 TO 20 MINUTES

One of my favorite snack foods as a kid was CornNuts. In junior high, I used to get in trouble for spending all my lunch money on multiple varieties from the cafeteria vending machine. But as I got older, my teeth just couldn't handle their too-tough chew. This roasted hominy recipe is a delightful alternative—crunchy on the outside and just tender enough on the inside. Tossed with my Aztec Spice Blend and a splash of lime, these tasty kernels will hit you with just the right amount of flavor.

2 (15½-ounce) cans hominy, drained, rinsed, and patted dry
1 tablespoon olive oil
1 to 2 tablespoons Aztec Spice Blend (page 229)

Juice of 1 lime
¼ teaspoon salt

1. Preheat the oven to 425°F. Line a baking sheet with parchment paper.

2. Toss all the ingredients in a large bowl, mixing well to coat the hominy.

3. Evenly spread the coated hominy on the baking sheet.

4. Roast for 15 to 20 minutes, stirring and turning the pan halfway through the cooking time.

COOKING TIP: Spice up any soup or salad with these spicy kernels. Use them as you would croutons for an Aztec-inspired twist.

ELOTES

SERVES 4 • PREP TIME: 10 MINUTES • COOK TIME: 20 MINUTES

If you've ever been to Mexico, or walked through any densely populated Mexican neighborhood in the US, you've probably heard someone selling elotes. Street vendors call out, "Elotes calientes . . . con limón, mayonesa, chile y queso!" Hungry residents and passersby quickly flock to the truck or cart for this super tasty treat. It's just like American-style corn on the cob—grilled to perfection—but Mexican-style elotes are coated with fresh lime juice, chili powder, and one of my favorite condiments: vegan mayo (I like Just Mayo). Sprinkle on some of my Almond Queso Cotija and you're in for a super tasty treat!

¼ cup vegan mayo
¼ cup Cashew Crema Mexicana (page 230)
1 teaspoon chili powder
¼ teaspoon garlic powder

1 chipotle in adobo, minced
4 ears fresh corn, husk on
¾ cup Almond Queso Cotija (page 73)
1 lime, quartered
Vinegar hot sauce, to taste

1. Heat a grill to 500°F. If you're using a wood or charcoal grill, heat until the coals are white hot.

2. In a small bowl, whisk together the mayo, Cashew Crema Mexicana, chili powder, and garlic powder. Add the minced chipotle and combine. Set aside.

3. Shuck the corn, leaving some of the husk intact to twist into a handle for grilling and to hold while eating.

4. Place the corn on the grill toward the end and let the twisted husk hang off the grill so it will not burn. Use the corn husks to rotate the corn every 2½ to 3 minutes, grilling the corn evenly on all sides. Total grill time should be about 10 minutes for a nice char on all sides.

5. Remove the corn from the grill and coat with the mayo-crema mixture and a generous coating of Almond Queso Cotija. Squeeze some lime on the corn and drizzle with your favorite vinegar hot sauce.

SECRET INGREDIENT: Vinegar hot sauce is a liquid hot chile sauce with a vinegar base—like Tabasco. There are hundreds of these, ranging from mild to crazy hot. Every region—seemingly worldwide—has their own. Valentina is my go-to brand for elotes.

COOKING TIP: No grill? Use a very hot cast-iron skillet and follow the same cooking instructions.

ALMOND QUESO COTIJA

MAKES 8 OUNCES • PREP TIME: 5 MINUTES

Cotija cheese was a staple in Casa Garza when I was growing up. We used it for everything—in place of Parmesan on pizza and as the perfect topper for popcorn. When you want a cheesy topping to accompany your dish but a sauce just isn't the right call, reach for this crumbly Almond Queso Cotija. Use it to top your enchiladas, sopes, elotes, and everything. Traditionally a seasonal cheese made up in the mountains of Michoacán, this super simple plant-based version can be made year-round in minutes—and at any altitude!

1 cup blanched almonds
1 teaspoon salt

½ teaspoon nutritional yeast
Juice of 1 lime

1. Pulse the almonds in a food processor until they have a texture that resembles crumbly Parmesan.

2. Transfer to a small mixing bowl and use your hands to combine with the salt, nutritional yeast, and lime juice.

3. Store in the refrigerator for up to 7 days.

COOKING TIP: Triple this recipe and use it on a variety of dishes, including salads and tacos, or to garnish just about any dish in this cookbook.

CASHEW QUESO FUNDIDO

SERVES 3 • PREP TIME: 10 MINUTES, PLUS 20 MINUTES SOAKING TIME •
COOK TIME: 10 MINUTES

*As an increasingly popular member of the cheesy dip family, Queso
Fundido wins the award for gooeyness! This combination of stretchy
cashew-tapioca cheese topped with spicy Garbanzorizo is sure to be a hit
as an appetizer or out on the spread at a casual gathering or cookout.
Spoon this northern Mexican delight onto warm, soft tortillas and enjoy!*

½ cup raw cashews, soaked in hot
    water for 20 minutes or boiled
    until soft
1 cup water
½ tablespoon nutritional yeast
3 tablespoons tapioca flour
1 teaspoon apple cider vinegar
½ teaspoon salt

½ teaspoon garlic powder
½ teaspoon mustard powder
¼ teaspoon white pepper
1 tablespoon olive oil
1 cup Garbanzorizo (page 242)
3 to 6 corn tortillas, warmed

1. Drain and rinse the cashews.

2. Toss the cashews, water, nutritional yeast, tapioca flour, vinegar, salt, garlic powder, mustard powder, and pepper into a blender. Blend until smooth and set aside.

3. Warm the oil in a small skillet and heat the Garbanzorizo just to warm it through.

4. Pour the cashew mixture into a small heavy-bottomed saucepan and cook over medium-high heat, stirring constantly with a wooden spoon. The mixture should start to get lumpy. After about 5 minutes, you will have a nice stretchy cheese.

5. Serve in a deep bowl and top with Garbanzorizo. Serve with warm corn tortillas.

COOKING TIP: Rinsing the cashews after soaking helps keep the cheese a nice bright white color.

CHILI SIN QUESO

MAKES 4 CUPS • PREP TIME: 10 MINUTES, PLUS 20 MINUTES SOAKING TIME •
COOK TIME: 35 MINUTES

*The last nonvegan meal I ever ate was at a restaurant in Dallas called
Gloria's. I'd been weaning myself off dairy for weeks and I planned my
last meal as a lacto-vegetarian to be my absolute favorite party snack:
chili con queso. Chili con queso can be made with any number of meltable
cheeses. For this vegan version, we're going for the classic Tex-Mex–style
I grew up with, featuring creamy butternut squash, cashews, and cheesy
nutritional yeast. Whether it is a movie night, party time, or if you are just
having a few friends and family over for dinner, Chili sin Queso is great as
a dip, over nachos, as a Mexican twist on mac and cheese, and more.*

½ cup raw cashews
1 small butternut squash, peeled,
   seeded and diced medium
3 garlic cloves
1 tablespoon olive oil
½ medium onion, diced
1 teaspoon ground cumin
1 teaspoon chili powder
1 to 2 teaspoons salt
1 chipotle in adobo

3 to 4 tablespoons nutritional yeast
2 tablespoons Dijon or spicy
   brown mustard
1 to 2 teaspoons apple cider vinegar
1 (10-ounce) can diced tomatoes with
   chiles, drained

GARNISH OPTIONS
Pico de Gallo (page 198)
Chopped cilantro

1. Soak the cashews in hot water for 20 minutes.

2. While they are soaking, place the butternut squash in a pot, cover with water, and boil about 20 minutes, or until soft. Add the garlic cloves for the last 10 minutes of cooking.

3. Preheat a skillet on medium heat and add the oil. Sauté the onion for 5 to 7 minutes. Add the cumin, chili powder, salt, and chipotle, and sauté for 2 more minutes. Remove from the heat.

4. When the squash is soft, drain the water, reserving about 2 cups for the sauce.

5. Add the squash, garlic, and some of the cooking liquid to a blender and purée. Add the soaked cashews and enough cooking liquid to keep the mixture moving. When the cashews are very smooth, add the spice and onion mixture and the nutritional yeast, mustard, and vinegar. Blend thoroughly. Add the tomatoes and chiles and pulse a few times to combine.

6. Top with the garnishes of your choice.

HEAT INDEX: Go for a spicy mustard; the bolder the mustard, the more pop the sauce will have.

NACHOS GRANDE

MAKES 1 LARGE PLATE • PREP TIME: 15 MINUTES • COOK TIME: 10 MINUTES

What Mexican cookbook would be complete without a nacho recipe? The now-ubiquitous dish is enjoyed at ballparks, movie theaters, and of course restaurants worldwide. This modern take on the now-classic snack food features a creamy butternut squash–based cheese and is loaded with black beans, corn, guacamole, and pico de gallo. Remember: Nachos are meant for sharing. And sharing is caring. As J.D. says in the movie Saving Silverman, *"If you get the nachos stuck together, that's one nacho."*

1 tablespoon vegetable oil
¼ cup corn kernels, fresh or frozen
Salt
Freshly ground black pepper
½ cup Refried Black Beans (page 171)
½ cup Chili sin Queso (page 75)

2 handfuls tortillas chips
¼ cup Classic Guacamole (page 235)
¼ cup Pico de Gallo (page 198)
1 tablespoon chopped cilantro
Drizzle of Cashew Crema
    Mexicana (page 230)

1. Heat a skillet on medium-high and add the oil. Add the corn and season with salt and pepper. Cook for 3 to 4 minutes, stirring occasionally, until the corn is nicely browned.

2. Meanwhile, reheat the Refried Black Beans and Chili sin Queso separately, on the stovetop or in the microwave.

3. Place the tortilla chips on a large plate and top with beans, chili, roasted corn, Classic Guacamole, Pico de Gallo, and cilantro. Drizzle with Cashew Crema Mexicana. Enjoy!

ORIGIN STORY: Nachos originated in northern Mexico, where, in 1943, Ignacio "Nacho" Anaya fried up a bunch of corn tortillas, covered them with Cheddar cheese, and topped the newly invented dish with sliced jalapeño chiles.

CLASSIC QUESADILLAS

MAKES 12 QUESADILLAS • PREP TIME: 20 MINUTES • COOK TIME: 20 MINUTES

Quesadillas are the perfect party food! They're easy to make and easy to serve, and everybody loves them. Like most traditional Mexican dishes, quesadillas have evolved many times since their original days in colonial Mexico. These days, there are countless variations across the world. At Garza gatherings, friends love pressing their own fresh masa discs, and I take care of toasting them made-to-order.

12 Handmade Corn Tortillas (page 232)
Nonstick cooking spray

3 cups shredded vegan white cheese
Red or green salsa

1. Prepare the Handmade Corn Tortillas according to the recipe.

2. Heat a large nonstick griddle or skillet to medium and lightly spray with non-stick cooking spray. Carefully peel the top sheet of waxed paper from a pressed Handmade Corn Tortilla. Place the disc directly onto the griddle (waxed paper facing up). Carefully peel the waxed paper from the tortilla, making sure not to tear the disc.

3. Spread ¼ cup of cheese evenly over the Handmade Corn Tortilla. Once the cheese starts to melt, fold the tortilla

in half and cook for about 1 minute more on each side, or until the cheese is melted and the tortilla is crispy on both sides.

4. Serve the quesadillas hot with a side of red or green salsa.

ORIGIN STORY: The quesadilla most Americans know and love is a large folded flour tortilla stuffed with gooey cheese and other hefty fillers, and is often cut into halves or quarters for easy sharing. This classic version from the colonial city of Leon, Guanajuato, is much smaller.

ZUCCHINI BLOSSOM QUESADILLAS

MAKES 12 QUESADILLAS • PREP TIME: 20 MINUTES • COOK TIME: 20 TO 25 MINUTES

On the edge of Mexico City is the beautiful national park Desierto de los Leones *(Desert of the Lions), where city residents often escape the hustle and bustle of city life for a hike. After getting lost in the sky-high pines and gorgeous waterfalls, hikers don't head back into the busy city streets without stopping by a nearby village where native folks cook up fresh zucchini blossom quesadillas. When cooked, zucchini blossoms release beautiful bright yellow dye and give these quesadillas a delicate, silky mouthfeel.*

2 cups corn masa flour
½ teaspoon salt
1½ cups warm water
Nonstick cooking spray
3 cups shredded vegan white cheese

24 small zucchini blossoms
  (2½ to 3 inches long), chopped
12 fresh epazote leaves, chopped
Red or green salsa, for serving

1. Cut twenty-four 8-by-12-inch sheets of waxed paper for the tortilla press.

2. In a large bowl, mix together the corn masa flour and salt. Add the water and combine.

3. Divide the masa into twelve equal portions and form into football-shaped masa rolls.

4. Line the bottom of the tortilla press with a sheet of waxed paper and place one masa roll in the center of the press. Cover the roll with another piece of waxed paper. Press the masa into a thin disc. Remove the masa disc, still between the waxed paper sheets, and set aside. Repeat until all the rolls have been pressed.

5. Heat a large nonstick griddle or skillet to medium and lightly spray with non-stick cooking spray. Carefully peel the top sheet of waxed paper from a pressed masa. Place the disc directly onto the griddle (waxed paper facing up). Carefully peel the waxed paper from the masa, making sure not to tear the disc.

6. Spread ¼ cup of cheese, 2 blossoms, and 1 epazote leaf evenly over the masa disc. Once the cheese starts to melt, fold the tortilla in half and cook for about 1 to 1½ minutes more on each side, or until the cheese is melted and the tortilla is crispy on both sides. Repeat with the other quesadillas.

7. Serve quesadillas hot with a side of red or green salsa, if desired.

SECRET INGREDIENT: Fresh epazote can be found at any Latin market. Fresh zucchini blossoms can be found at many natural grocers, and canned blossoms can be found at most Latin markets. If you can't find zucchini blossoms or fresh epazote, use thin slices of zucchini and chopped cilantro instead.

COOKING TIP: If you don't have a tortilla press, don't stress. Line a cutting board with waxed paper, place a masa roll in the center, and cover with another piece of waxed paper. Press the masa with a large, heavy hardcover book, such as a dictionary or encyclopedia.

BLACK BEAN AND GUACAMOLE SOPES

MAKES 4 • PREP TIME: 25 MINUTES • COOK TIME: 10 MINUTES

On May 7, 1983, I had my very first sope. It was my sixth birthday and I remember the day like it was yesterday. My dad had walked my brother Michael and me across the bridge to Matamoros, Mexico, where we celebrated my special day at the Mercado Juárez, at a hole-in-the-wall restaurant my dad swore made the best sopes. One taste and I was in love. We ordered sopes for appetizers, then I ordered seconds as my birthday meal. The base of any great sope is a perfectly formed corn boat. This sopes recipe is the perfect balance of tender and crispy, piled high with spicy refried beans, guacamole, fresh lettuce, and red onion, then topped Almond Queso Cotija. ¡Que rico!

4 Handmade Sopes (page 234)
8 tablespoons Refried Black Beans
   (page 171)
4 tablespoons Classic Guacamole
   (page 235)
¾ to 1 cup shredded lettuce

4 teaspoons red onion, diced
4 tablespoons Almond Queso
   Cotija (page 73)

GARNISH OPTIONS
Red salsa of your choice
Vinegar hot sauce

1. Heat the Handmade Sopes on a large skillet or griddle. Place on 4 plates.

2. Fill each Handmade Sope with 2 tablespoons of Refried Black Beans, and top with 1 tablespoon of Classic Guacamole, some shredded lettuce, and 1 teaspoon of diced onion. Drizzle with 1 tablespoon of Almond Queso Cotija. Repeat until you've made all the sopes.

3. Serve with the garnishes of your choice.

ORIGIN STORY: Sopes—palm-size deep-dish corn cakes—originated in the northwestern Mexican city of Culiacán. You can make them yourself or buy them prepackaged at any Latin grocer.

SEAFOOD-STYLE ALBONDIGAS

MAKES 10 CAKES • PREP TIME: 15 MINUTES • COOK TIME: 20 MINUTES

If you like crab cakes, you're going to love these seafood albondigas! Albondiga means "meatball." Fondly referred to as Mexican soul food, albondigas' history dates back to the eighth century, when Islamic influence dominated in southwestern Europe. When the Spanish took over the region, many of the previous culinary traditions were integrated into Spanish cuisine. From there, albondigas made their way to Mexico by way of the conquistadors, where they have flourished into a cultural favorite.

2 tablespoons flaxseed

3 tablespoons water

1 (14-ounce) can hearts of palm, drained, cut in half lengthwise and sliced into 2-inch strips

1 (15.5-ounce) can garbanzo beans, drained, rinsed, and mashed

½ teaspoon ground cumin

¼ teaspoon garlic powder

1 teaspoon dulse flakes

¼ teaspoon freshly ground black pepper

¼ teaspoon salt

1 large baked russet potato, flesh scooped out and slightly mashed

Oil for frying

Lime wedges

Roasted Tomatillo Salsa (page 201)

1. In a small bowl, mix the flaxseed with the water and set aside.

2. In a large bowl, use your hands to mix the hearts of palm, mashed garbanzos, cumin, garlic powder, dulse, pepper, and salt, gently breaking up the hearts of palm. Fold the baked potato and the flaxseed into the hearts of palm–garbanzo mixture, and combine. The mix should be very rough and chunky.

3. Pour ¼ inch of oil in a large skillet and heat. Scoop up ¼ cup of the mixture and carefully slide it into the hot oil. Fry for 5 to 7 minutes on each side. Work in batches, if necessary, topping up the oil to keep it at ¼ inch. After frying, drain the cakes on paper towels and pat dry.

4. Give each a generous squeeze of lime and a pinch of salt. Serve with Roasted Tomatillo Salsa.

COOKING TIP: These albondigas are the base for the Baja Burrito with Mango Salsa (page 204), but you can also use leftover albondigas to make crabcake-style sandwiches. Simply lather a standard burger bun with vegan chipotle mayo and top with lettuce and tomato for a quick and easy meal.

PAPAS BRAVAS

SERVES 4 • PREP TIME: 10 MINUTES • COOK TIME: 40 TO 60 MINUTES

In Mexico, I've often seen papas bravas, a spicy potato dish, prepared as wedges and served as a side dish with tortas and other sandwiches—sort of like home fries. But these papas bravas should be a sidekick to no dish; they deserve a spotlight of their own. When I make these for tapas parties at Casa Garza, they're always the first thing to disappear. For a really nice presentation, use tricolored peewee potatoes.

FOR THE POTATOES
1 pound red potatoes or
    Yukon golds, unpeeled,
    cut into ¼-inch wedges
2 tablespoons olive oil
1 teaspoon Aztec Spice
    Blend (page 229)

FOR THE SAUCE
1 teaspoon vegetable oil
2 garlic cloves, minced
½ onion, diced small

½ teaspoon Aztec Spice
    Blend (page 229)
¼ teaspoon dried Mexican oregano
1 teaspoon Classic Chile
    Paste (page 194)
1 (15-ounce) can diced tomatoes,
    not drained
1 (4-ounce) can tomato sauce
1 to 2 teaspoons apple cider vinegar

TO GARNISH
Red onion, diced
Cilantro, chopped

1. TO MAKE THE POTATOES: Preheat the oven to 400°F. Line a baking sheet with parchment paper.

2. In a large mixing bowl, coat the potatoes with the oil and Aztec Spice Blend, and mix well.

3. Spread the potatoes evenly on the baking sheet. Roast for 40 minutes to an hour, stirring halfway through. While they are roasting, make the sauce.

1. TO MAKE THE SAUCE: Warm the oil in a large skillet and sauté the garlic on medium-high heat for 3 to 5 minutes.

2. Add the onion, Aztec Spice Blend, oregano, and Classic Chile Paste, and stir.

3. Add the tomatoes and their juice and the tomato sauce and simmer for 15 to 20 minutes. Use the vinegar to adjust for the tartness or sweetness of the tomatoes.

4. Purée the sauce with an immersion blender or in a blender.

5. Place the potatoes in a large serving bowl, sauce them generously, and garnish with red onion and cilantro.

Papas bravas is a great example of Spanish influence in Mexican cuisine. In Spain, they're called *patatas bravas* and are most commonly prepared like home fries and served as a small plate before dinner. You can find them at pretty much every tapas bar across the country.

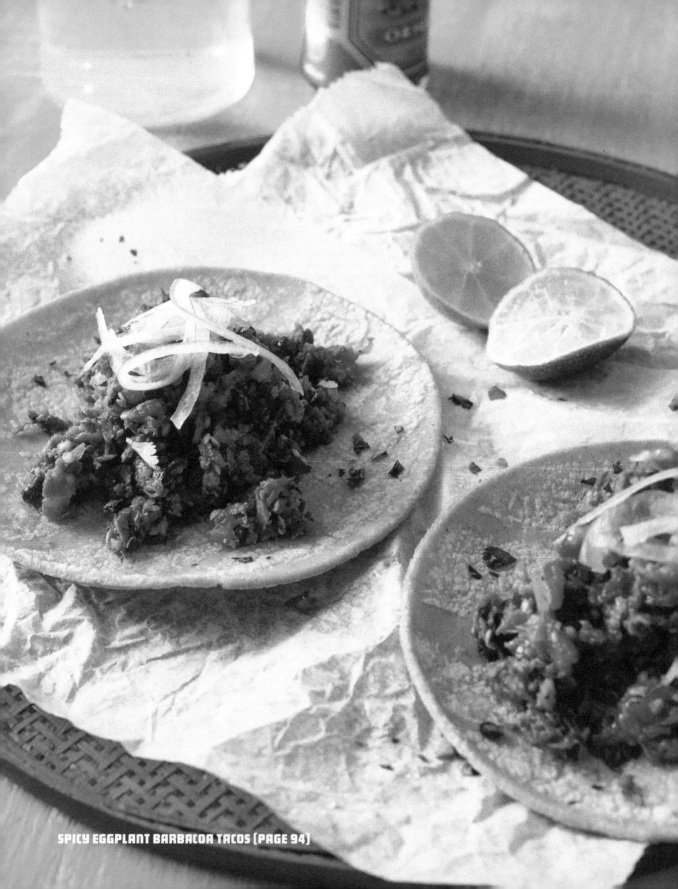

SPICY EGGPLANT BARBACOA TACOS (PAGE 94)

Chapter 5

TACOS, TORTAS, AND TAMALES

TACOS DE SUADERO

MAKES 8 TACOS • PREP TIME: 10 MINUTES • COOK TIME: 10 MINUTES

On the streets of most densely populated Mexican cities, you'll see taco stands on practically every corner. One of the most popular offerings you'll find are Tacos de Suadero, which are traditionally made with meat from between the rear leg and stomach of a cow. At Mexico City's Por Siempre Vegana Taquería and Monterrey's La Oveja Verde—two all-vegan taquerías—you'll find delicious soy-based versions of this popular dish. Once your tacos are piled high with soy meat, you'll be asked "con todo?"—"with everything?" (That means finely diced onion and cilantro.) Of course, the only correct answer is an enthusiastic "¡Sí!" My Tacos de Suadero are made with savory seared seitan, and the best way to enjoy them is definitely con todo.

1 tablespoon vegetable oil
1 pound Mexican Seasoned Seitan
    (page 239), chopped
3 garlic cloves, minced
¼ teaspoon salt
½ teaspoon freshly ground
    black pepper

8 corn tortillas, warmed
1 medium onion, diced
½ bunch cilantro, chopped
2 limes, quartered

1. Heat the oil in a large skillet on medium-high heat. Sauté the chopped Mexican Seasoned Seitan and garlic for 5 to 7 minutes. It will get a nice brown sear on it and have some crunchy bits on the ends.

2. Mix with the salt and pepper.

3. Serve on warm tortillas with generous amounts of onion and cilantro. Serve each plate with 2 lime wedges.

COOKING TIP: You can use leftover suadero filling in more than just tacos. Try it tossed in with Migas (page 38), or as a meaty topper for sopes.

COOKING TIP: This recipe takes only 20 minutes if you have the seitan already prepared.

TACOS AL PASTOR

MAKES 8 TACOS • PREP TIME: 20 MINUTES, PLUS 1 HOUR MARINATING TIME •
COOK TIME: 15 MINUTES

When I was a kid, nearly every weekend my family and I would walk across the B&M International Bridge to feast on the street tacos in Matamoros, Mexico. Nine times out of ten, I ordered Tacos al Pastor—pineapple and chile-rubbed shawarma-style tacos that were made popular by Lebanese immigrants to Mexico who incorporated local ingredients into their cooking methods. Fusion food at its finest!

FOR THE MARINADE
2 cups fresh pineapple, peeled
   and diced
4 chipotle chiles in adobo, plus
   3 tablespoons of the adobo sauce
   from the can
¼ cup fresh lime juice
3 garlic cloves, minced
½ cup diced white onion
1 teaspoon dried Mexican oregano
1 teaspoon freshly ground black pepper
1 teaspoon achiote paste or powder

1 teaspoon ground cumin
¼ teaspoon salt

FOR THE TACOS
1 pound Mexican Seasoned Seitan
   (page 239), chopped
1 tablespoon vegetable oil
8 corn tortillas
1½ cups diced fresh pineapple
1 medium onion, diced
½ bunch chopped cilantro

1. TO MAKE THE MARINADE: Place all the ingredients in a blender and blend for about 3 minutes. It can still have some pieces of pineapple that are not completely smooth.

2. Pour over the chopped seitan and marinate for at least 1 hour. Discard the marinade.

1. TO MAKE THE TACOS: Heat the oil in a large skillet on medium-high heat. Sauté the marinated seitan for 5 to 10 minutes, stirring frequently. The mixture will have a deep red color and will be quite

spicy. Cook the seitan until it browns well, adjusting the heat as needed. The sugar in the pineapple can caramelize, so watch it very carefully.

2. Remove the marinated seitan from the heat and serve on warm corn tortillas with fresh pineapple, onion, and cilantro.

HEAT INDEX: Too hot to handle? Simply omit the chipotles from the marinade and add 1 tablespoon smoked paprika. You'll get the same beautiful red color and smoky flavor without the heat.

GREEN CHORIZO TACOS

MAKES 8 TACOS • PREP TIME: 10 MINUTES • COOK TIME: 10 MINUTES

Green seitan chorizo is the star of these uniquely inspired tacos! The city of Toluca is famous for its wide variety of chorizo offerings, with green chorizo being a specialty. My version of Toluca's green chorizo tacos is an environmentally friendly twist on this Mexican favorite!

1 tablespoon olive oil
½ medium onion, sliced thin
2 pounds Green Seitan Chorizo (page 240), chopped up like ground sausage
8 corn tortillas
½ medium onion, diced small

¼ bunch cilantro, chopped
½ cup Cashew Crema Mexicana (page 230)
½ cup Roasted Tomatillo Salsa (page 201)
2 limes, quartered

1. Heat the oil in a large skillet on medium-high heat. Sauté the sliced onion for 3 to 5 minutes. Add the Green Seitan Chorizo and sauté for another 7 minutes, or until nicely browned.

2. Serve on warm corn tortillas with diced onion and cilantro. Drizzle with Cashew Crema Mexicana and Roasted Tomatillo Salsa. Serve with lime wedges.

COOKING TIP: Use this sausage on the grill and make a Toluca, a Mexican-inspired East Coast–style grinder with peppers, onion, and some shredded cheese on a hoagie roll.

TACOS DE NOPALES

MAKES 8 TACOS • PREP TIME: 10 MINUTES • COOK TIME: 15 MINUTES

Sporting sharp thorns, cactus plants might not appear edible at first. But they've been a fundamental part of the Mexican diet for thousands of years. Throughout Mexico and the American Southwest, nopal cactus is a ridiculously popular vegetable, and for good reason: It's considered a superfood, thanks to its antioxidants and cholesterol-reducing properties. It's the star ingredient in these tacos, prepared in the Central Mexico style—sautéed with savory onions, garlic, and cilantro, then sprinkled with Almond Queso Cotija. ¡Delicioso!

1 teaspoon vegetable oil
1 medium onion, thinly sliced
3 garlic cloves, minced
24 nopal cactus pads, dethorned, peeled, and sliced
¼ teaspoon salt
¼ teaspoon freshly ground black pepper

8 corn tortillas
½ bunch cilantro, chopped
8 tablespoons Almond Queso Cotija (page 73)
2 limes, quartered

1. Heat the oil in a large skillet on medium-high heat. Sauté the onion for 3 to 5 minutes. It is okay if it gets some color, as it will add a nice sweetness to the dish.

2. Add the garlic and nopales and sauté for 7 to 10 more minutes. The cactus should still be somewhat firm when finished. Mix with the salt and pepper.

3. Serve on warm corn tortillas and top with cilantro and Almond Queso Cotija. Serve with lime wedges.

SECRET INGREDIENT: Head to a Latin market for budget-friendly nopales and you'll save a lot of time. These cactus pads are often sold prewashed, sliced, and ready to cook.

BAJA TACOS

MAKES 12 TACOS • PREP TIME: 20 MINUTES • COOK TIME: 20 MINUTES

Surrounded by the sea, the peninsula of Baja California is well-known for its sun, surf, and fish tacos. There's vigorous debate over which port town originated the tacos, but one thing's clear: They're a big part of the Baja California experience. My vegan Baja Tacos—with a crunchy beer-battered outside (I like Modelo Especial or Tecate) and soft cauliflower inside—are a perfect alternative to those fried fish bits. Top them with fresh red cabbage, avocado, pico de gallo, and spicy chipotle mayo, and you'll feel like the sun and surf are right there with you.

FOR THE BATTER
2½ cups white rice flour
2 teaspoons baking powder
1 teaspoon ground cumin
1 teaspoon chili powder
1 teaspoon garlic powder
½ teaspoon salt
½ teaspoon freshly ground
   black pepper
2 (12-ounce) bottles of Mexican lager
1 head cauliflower, cut into
   bite-size florets

FOR THE TACOS
4 cups vegetable oil, for frying
Salt
12 corn tortillas
2 cups red cabbage, julienned
1 cup vegan chipotle mayo
2 avocados, peeled and sliced
2 cups Pico de Gallo (page 198)

1. **TO MAKE THE BATTER:** In a large bowl, whisk together the rice flour, baking powder, cumin, chili powder, garlic powder, salt, and pepper.

2. Pour in 1½ bottles of beer and whisk well. The batter should resemble a slightly thick pancake batter. If it's too thick, add a little bit more beer to loosen the batter. Use right away.

3. Toss the cauliflower into the batter and coat well by mixing it with your hands.

1. **TO MAKE THE TACOS:** Heat the oil in a large pot on medium heat to 350°F. Use a thermometer to check the temperature.

2. When the oil has reached the right temperature, carefully drop in a few pieces of cauliflower, one at a time, and cook 3 to 4 minutes each. When the

pieces are nicely browned, remove with tongs and place on a heat-resistant paper towel–lined plate, or a roasting rack, to allow excess oil to drip. You might need to increase the heat to keep the oil at a constant temperature. Repeat until all the cauliflower is cooked. Lightly sprinkle the fried bits with salt.

3. To build the tacos, place 3 to 5 cauliflower florets in the center of each tortilla. Top each taco with a pinch of shredded cabbage, a dollop of the chipotle mayo, sliced avocado, and some Pico de Gallo. Repeat to make all the tacos.

COOKING TIP: If you prefer a lower-fat or nonalcoholic version, mix the rice flour, baking powder, cumin, chili powder, garlic powder, salt, and pepper with 2 tablespoons of olive oil, toss with the cauliflower to coat, and roast in a 400°F oven for 20 minutes.

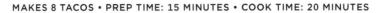

SPICY EGGPLANT BARBACOA TACOS

MAKES 8 TACOS • PREP TIME: 15 MINUTES • COOK TIME: 20 MINUTES

In the cattle ranching regions of Mexico, barbacoa is typically made with meat from a cow's head—the eyes, cheek, brains, and more. The combination of the mostly unwanted parts gives the meat a texture unlike any other. Since going vegan, I've been on a mission to find a good alternative to this traditional Sunday morning meal at Casa Garza. Enter eggplant. A longtime star in the vegan culinary scene, eggplant's versatility really shines in these perfectly textured ranch-style tacos.

2 eggplants, shredded on the large holes of a box grater

3 cups water

Juice of 2 limes

1¼ teaspoons salt, divided, plus more for seasoning

1 tablespoon vegetable oil

1 medium white onion, diced, divided

3 garlic cloves, minced

1 fresh chile de árbol or serrano chile, seeded and minced

1 tablespoon ground cumin

1 teaspoon dark chili powder

½ teaspoon dried Mexican oregano

½ teaspoon chipotle powder

½ teaspoon freshly ground black pepper, plus more for seasoning

1 (15-ounce) can diced tomatoes, drained

8 corn tortillas

¼ cup chopped cilantro

2 limes, quartered

1. Soak the shredded eggplant in the water with the lime juice and 1 teaspoon of salt for 5 to 7 minutes. Drain and squeeze out the excess water.

2. Heat the oil in a large skillet on medium-high heat. Sauté half the onion with the garlic and chile de árbol or serrano chile for 3 to 4 minutes. Add the cumin, chili powder, oregano, chipotle powder, pepper, and remaining ¼ teaspoon salt, and sauté for 2 more minutes.

3. Add the shredded eggplant and cook for 10 to 15 minutes, stirring as needed. You want the eggplant to cook out some of the liquid and brown slightly. In the last 5 minutes of cooking, add the tomatoes and season again with salt and pepper.

4. Serve on warm corn tortillas with the rest of the chopped onion and cilantro. Serve with lime wedges.

COOKING TIP: This barbacoa recipe is also great as burrito bowl topper. Serve over a bed of Cilantro Lime Rice (page 162) and top with Pico de Gallo (page 198), Classic Guacamole (page 235), Almond Queso Cotija (page 73), and a handful of shredded romaine lettuce.

CHICKEN-STYLE SETAS TACOS

MAKES 8 TACOS • PREP TIME: 10 MINUTES, PLUS 1 HOUR MARINATING TIME • COOK TIME: 15 MINUTES

Seared oyster mushrooms are the star of these delicious tacos. I often use oyster mushrooms as an alternative to chicken because of their soft texture and ability to capture the robust flavors of blackened or grilled chicken. The trick is to lather the mushrooms with olive oil and my Aztec Rub and marinate for at least an hour before searing. The end result is a smoky taco plate even the most fervent carnivore will love.

2 pounds oyster mushrooms
4 tablespoons olive oil, divided
2 to 3 tablespoons Aztec Spice Blend
  (page 229)

1 medium onion, ½ julienned,
  ½ diced small
8 corn tortillas
½ bunch cilantro, chopped
2 limes, quartered

1. In a large bowl, toss the oyster mushrooms with 3 tablespoons of olive oil and the Aztec Spice Blend. Set aside to marinate 1 to 4 hours.

2. Preheat a large cast-iron skillet on medium-high heat. Add 1 tablespoon of oil and the mushrooms, and press down with a second skillet (or a steak weight grill press, if you have one). This is a fast-sear method, so both pans get extremely hot. Be careful not to burn yourself or the mushrooms. Sear the mushrooms for about 3 to 5 minutes, turn them over, and press again. Reduce the heat to medium and cook 5 more minutes.

3. Remove the mushrooms from the pan and let them rest 2 to 3 minutes. They should have a nice charred look to them.

4. In the same hot pan, add the julienned onion and just a tad more oil and sauté for 2 to 3 minutes. Remove from the heat. Slice or pull the mushrooms apart and mix with both the sautéed onions.

5. To build the tacos, serve on warm corn tortillas with the diced onions, cilantro, and lime wedges.

COOKING TIP: If fast-searing sounds like a frightening task, try an outdoor grill instead. Marinate the mushrooms and grill on a direct flame for 7 minutes on each side. Another option is to roast them in the oven at 425°F for 20 to 30 minutes, stirring halfway through.

GRINGO TACOS

MAKES 4 TACOS • PREP TIME: 10 MINUTES • COOK TIME: 15 MINUTES

If you think traditions are meant to be broken, then I have a taco for you! "Gringo" tacos might appear to be your average taco, but they break from tradition in that they call for a large flour tortilla instead of a small corn tortilla. Then, breaking another tradition, they are packed with multiple ingredients. This taco features refried black beans, seared oyster mushrooms, sautéed onions, poblano chiles, guacamole, and pico de gallo. Taco stands all over Mexico are adding gringo tacos to their menus, and now so can you!

¾ cup Refried Black Beans (page 171)
1 tablespoon olive oil
1 poblano chile, seeded
   and julienned
1 medium white onion, julienned
¼ teaspoon salt
¼ teaspoon freshly ground
   black pepper

1 pound Seared Chicken-Style Setas
   (page 238)
4 (6-inch) flour tortillas
1 cup Classic Guacamole (page 235)
½ cup Pico de Gallo (page 198)

1. In a small saucepan (or a microwave), heat the Refried Black Beans on medium heat until warm, and set aside.

2. Heat the oil in a large skillet on medium-high heat and the sauté the poblano chile and onion for 5 to 7 minutes. Sprinkle with the salt and pepper. Add the Seared Chicken-Style Setas and sauté for 3 to 4 minutes more, until heated through.

3. To build the tacos, smear a couple of tablespoons of beans on a tortilla, then top with the mushroom and onion mixture. Top with the Classic Guacamole and Pico de Gallo, and enjoy.

ORIGIN STORY: In Mexico, the word *gringo* refers to someone from the United States. The name of this taco comes from the idea that flour tortillas are preferred north of the Mexican border.

REFRIED BEAN AND SEITAN BEEF-STYLE TOSTADAS

MAKES 4 TOSTADAS • PREP TIME: 20 TO 25 MINUTES • COOK TIME: 20 MINUTES

Tostadas are corn tortillas that have been deep fried or toasted, then lathered with refried beans, which keep the other toppings from falling off. This northern Mexican–style tostada features spicy refried pinto beans, chopped seitan beef, then topped with shredded lettuce, tomato, and vegan Cheddar cheese. They're perfect for sharing as a starter with friends or as a full entrée for yourself.

1 cup Spicy Refried Pinto Beans
 (page 174)
1 cup vegetable oil, for frying
4 corn tortillas
1 cup chopped Mexican Seasoned
 Seitan (page 239)
1 teaspoon olive oil
1 chipotle chile, minced
1 teaspoon ground cumin
1 teaspoon garlic powder

½ teaspoon freshly ground
 black pepper
¼ teaspoon salt
1 cup chopped green leaf or
 iceberg lettuce
2 Roma tomatoes, diced small
4 radishes, sliced
1 cup vegan shredded Cheddar or
 pepper Jack cheese

1. Warm the Spicy Refried Pinto Beans in a small saucepan (or a microwave) on medium heat until hot. Set aside.

2. Heat the vegetable oil in a large skillet on medium-high heat and fry the tortillas until they are brown and crispy, about 1 minute per side. Let rest on paper towels to drain the excess oil. Pour most of the remaining oil into a safe dish for cooling.

3. In the same pan, sauté the Mexican Seasoned Seitan in olive oil for about 3 minutes. Add the chipotle chile, cumin, garlic powder, black pepper, and salt, and sauté for another 5 minutes. Remove from the heat.

4. To build the tostadas, smear some Spicy Refried Pinto Beans on the tortilla and top with the Mexican Seasoned Seitan, lettuce, tomatoes, radishes, and cheese.

COOKING TIP: To cut some calories, you can bake the tortillas instead of frying them. Preheat your oven to 400°F, lightly brush the tortillas with oil on each side, then place them on a baking sheet and bake for 3 to 5 minutes per side, until they're just crispy.

SEITAN BISTEC TORTAS

MAKES 4 TORTAS • PREP TIME: 10 MINUTES • COOK TIME: 15 MINUTES

Bistec torta means "steak sandwich" in Spanish. It's typically made with thinly sliced, tenderized skirt steak. This vegan version of a Garza family favorite features a tender seitan steak instead. Seared to perfection and topped with crisp lettuce, onion, and creamy avocado, this hearty sandwich will please your entire family.

2 tablespoons olive oil
1 pound Mexican Seasoned Seitan
   (page 239), thinly sliced
1 teaspoon garlic powder
½ teaspoon ground cumin
¼ teaspoon dried Mexican oregano
¼ teaspoon salt
1 medium white onion, julienned

2 serrano chiles, sliced
2 large tomatoes, diced medium
Juice of 1 lime
4 tablespoons vegan chipotle mayo
4 bolillos, cut open and toasted
1 cup iceberg lettuce, shredded
1 avocado, peeled and smashed
¼ bunch cilantro, chopped

1. Heat the oil in a large skillet on medium-high heat. Sauté the Mexican Seasoned Seitan for 3 to 5 minutes. Add the garlic powder, cumin, oregano, and salt, and sauté for 2 minutes more.

2. When the seitan is well-browned, add the onion and serrano chiles and sauté for 3 more minutes. Add the tomatoes and heat through. Add the lime juice and remove from the heat.

3. To build the tortas, smear 1 tablespoon of mayo on the bottom half of each bolillo. Place ¼ of the seitan filling on top of the mayo, then stuff the torta with lettuce, avocado, and cilantro.

SIMPLE SWAP: Ditch the mayo and lettuce and top with melty vegan mozzarella for a Mexican twist on a Philly cheesesteak. Just make sure you keep the avocado!

JACKFRUIT CARNITAS TORTAS

MAKES 4 TORTAS • PREP TIME: 5 MINUTES • COOK TIME: 15 MINUTES

Jackfruit is used to create this carnitas-style torta. Jackfruit might be new to some regions of the world, but people in Latin America have been using this crop for centuries. Loved for its juicy mouthfeel and versatility, this tree fruit is filled with nutrients. It's a tasty source of protein, potassium, and vitamin A. This shredded meaty torta is perfectly complemented by avocado and Red Onion, Radish, and Cilantro Relish.

1 tablespoon olive oil
1 medium white onion, julienned
2 garlic cloves, minced
1 teaspoon ground cumin
½ teaspoon chipotle powder
¼ teaspoon salt
¼ teaspoon freshly ground
   black pepper

1 pound unseasoned prepackaged
   jackfruit, diced medium
1 tablespoon vegan butter
Juice of 1 lime
4 tablespoons vegan chipotle mayo
4 bolillos, cut open and toasted
1 avocado, peeled and sliced
4 tablespoons Red Onion, Radish,
   and Cilantro Relish (page 205)

1. To make the carnitas, heat the oil in a large skillet over medium-high heat. Sauté the onion and garlic for 3 minutes. Add the cumin, chipotle powder, salt, and pepper, and stir. Then add the jackfruit and sauté for 7 to 10 minutes, allowing the jackfruit to caramelize with the onion. As you stir, break the fruit apart to create shreds.

2. Add the butter and lime juice and stir constantly so the butter melts. Remove from the heat.

3. To build the tortas, spread 1 table-spoon of mayo on the bottom of each bolillo and spoon the carnitas on the bread. Top with sliced avocado and Red Onion, Radish, and Cilantro Relish.

SECRET INGREDIENT: Jackfruit can be found fresh, canned, or frozen in most Asian markets. If you buy canned jack-fruit, make sure to get the variety packed in water, not in syrup. Upton's Naturals Original Jackfruit, which comes in a vacuum pouch already shredded, is a great choice. If you buy a fresh one, pick a green jackfruit and search the Web for a host of tips and videos on cutting and seeding it.

COOKING TIP: If you have the salsa on hand, this recipes takes just 20 minutes start to finish.

BLACK BEAN BURGUESA TORTAS

MAKES 4 TORTAS • PREP TIME: 15 MINUTES • COOK TIME: 20 MINUTES

Let's face it: Everyone loves a good burger. That's why it should come as no surprise that even in Mexico you can chow down on an American-style burger with a Latin twist—a "burguesa" torta, if you will.

FOR THE BURGER
1 (15-ounce) can black beans, drained and rinsed
1 (12-ounce) can diced tomatoes, not drained
1 (4-ounce) can diced green chiles
2 tablespoons granulated garlic
1 tablespoon ground cumin
1 tablespoon chili powder
1 teaspoon salt
1 teaspoon freshly ground black pepper
3 tablespoons flaxseed mixed with ½ cup warm water, or egg replacer equivalent to 3 eggs

1 cup quick oats
Nonstick cooking spray

FOR THE TORTA
Vegan chipotle mayo
4 bolillos, cut open and toasted
1 large tomato, cut into 6 slices
1 small white onion, sliced
Pickled jalapeños
Classic Guacamole (page 235)

1. TO MAKE THE BURGERS: Using a food processor, pulse all the burger ingredients except the oats until well blended. Fold in quick oats and combine. The mixture should be somewhat wet and a little chunky.

2. If you don't have a food processor, no worries. Just mash the beans, tomatoes and their juice, and chiles with a fork, then add everything except the oats and combine with your hands. Add the oats last, and mix until well combined.

3. Form into 4 large patties.

4. Heat a griddle or skillet to medium-high and lightly spray with nonstick cooking spray. Cook the patties for about 7 minutes each side, or until well-browned. The crunchy browned outside will help keep the burgers together when you bite into them.

1. TO MAKE THE TORTAS: Spread some mayo on the bottom of each bolillo, then top with a burguesa patty, tomato, onion, and pickled jalapeños.

2. Lather the top of the bolillo with Classic Guacamole and enjoy.

COOKING TIP: My personal favorite way to cook these patties is to use an electric griddle, preheated to 375°F, so I can cook them all at once.

GRILLED VEGETABLE TORTAS

MAKES 4 TORTAS • PREP TIME: 15 MINUTES • COOK TIME: 10 MINUTES

Squashes of all kinds have been cultivated in Mexico since the Aztec and Maya eras. Some are used primarily for their seeds. Others could be hollowed out and used to make water containers. Some were devoured whole! As further proof of squashes' versatility and endurance through changes in cuisine over the years, nowadays we're grilling zucchini and summer squash with my signature Aztec Spice Rub; they can be eaten in a post-Mesoamerican–style torta.

1 medium zucchini, thinly cut on a bias
1 medium yellow squash, thinly cut
   on a bias
2 tablespoons olive oil
1 tablespoon Aztec Spice Blend
   (page 229)
½ medium white onion, julienned

1 poblano chile, seeded
   and julienned
4 bolillos, cut open and toasted
4 tablespoons vegan mayo
8 tablespoons Classic Guacamole
   (page 235)
2 Roma tomatoes, sliced thin
½ bunch cilantro, chopped

1. In a large bowl, toss the zucchini and squash with the oil and Aztec Spice Blend.

2. Heat a cast-iron grill pan on high heat and grill the squash slices for 3 to 4 minutes on each side. They should still have a nice crunch, but also have a good char to them. Remove from the heat and transfer to a bowl or plate.

3. Toss the onion and poblano chile in the same hot pan and cook for about 3 to 5 minutes, stirring occasionally with a wooden spoon. Reduce the heat if they start to burn before softening.

4. Put the grilled squash back in the pan, remove from the heat, and mix to combine.

5. To build the tortas, spread some mayo on the bottom of each bolillo. Fill each torta with equal amounts of the squash mixture. Spread Classic Guacamole on the top part of the roll. Top the grilled veggies with tomato slices and cilantro, and smash the torta shut with your hands.

SIMPLE SWAP: Use this recipe to try an assortment of summer squashes, like crookneck and zephyr squashes. Try roasting butternut squash and veggies such as Brussels sprouts for a warm fall torta.

JACKFRUIT GUISADO TORTAS

MAKES 6 TORTAS • PREP TIME: 10 MINUTES • COOK TIME: 45 MINUTES

One of my brother's and my favorite ways to enjoy Grandma's slow-simmered pulled pork growing up was in a toasted bolillo roll. It was our version of sloppy joes at Casa Garza. The trick is to slice the bolillos in half and toast the soft side just enough to hold up to the juicy filling. Top with avocado slices and fresh cilantro, and enjoy!

6 guajillo chiles, seeded
2 tablespoons vegetable oil, divided
½ medium onion, diced
3 garlic cloves, minced
1 (15-ounce) can diced tomatoes, not drained
1 chipotle chile, canned in adobo
1 teaspoon dried Mexican oregano
1 teaspoon ground cumin
¾ teaspoon chipotle powder

Salt
Freshly ground black pepper
Juice of 1 lime
1⅓ pounds prepared jackfruit (about two 10.6-ounce packages), chopped small
6 bolillos, sliced open and toasted
1 avocado, peeled, seeded, and sliced
¼ bunch cilantro, chopped

1. Toast the guajillo chiles on medium heat in a dry sauté pan until fragrant, about 5 minutes. Do not brown them.

2. In a small saucepan, heat 1 tablespoon vegetable oil over medium-high heat. Add the onion, garlic, and toasted guajillos. Sauté for 5 minutes, or until the onions are softened. Add the diced tomatoes and their juice, chipotle, oregano, cumin, chipotle powder, and season with salt and pepper. Simmer for 10 minutes.

3. Transfer the contents of saucepan to a blender. Add the lime juice and blend until smooth.

4. Heat the remaining 1 tablespoon of vegetable oil on high heat in a skillet and add the chopped jackfruit. Sauté to brown the jackfruit evenly. Pour the sauce from the blender over the jackfruit. Simmer until the sauce is reduced by about half, about 30 minutes.

5. Fill each bolillo with about 1 cup of the guisado. Garnish with avocado slices and cilantro. Press the torta shut with your hands.

COOKING TIP: Just like sloppy joes, these tortas are delightfully messy to eat, so make sure to have plenty of napkins on hand.

COCONUT AND PINEAPPLE CEVICHE TOSTADAS

MAKES 8 TOSTADAS • PREP TIME: 20 MINUTES, PLUS 1 HOUR CHILLING TIME • COOK TIME: 10 MINUTES

Ceviche tostadas are a popular dish along coastal regions of Mexico and throughout Latin America. They're typically made with raw seafood cured in lime juice, then blended with a mix of fruits and vegetables. Growing up, my dad used to make ceviche tostadas from raw oysters he picked from the bay of our neighboring town of Port Isabel, Texas. This modern take on one of my childhood favorites features young coconut meat, which does a fantastic job mimicking the texture of oysters. Crisp red onion and cucumber add a nice crunch, while fresh pineapple brings a welcome sweetness to the otherwise tart dish.

Meat of 3 young coconuts, chopped
    into small pieces (about ½ cup total)
1 cup diced fresh pineapple
1 large cucumber, peeled and
    diced small
½ cup diced red onion
1 medium serrano chile, seeded
    and chopped
1 to 2 tablespoons cilantro leaves

½ tablespoon olive oil
Juice of 1 lime
½ large Hass avocado, peeled
    and diced
¼ teaspoon salt
8 corn tortillas, toasted and
    broken into pieces

1. In a large mixing bowl, combine the coconut meat, pineapple, cucumber, onion, serrano chile, and cilantro. Mix well.

2. Add the olive oil and lime juice and combine.

3. Add the avocado and salt and toss gently.

4. Chill for at least 1 hour before serving.

5. Serve with toasted tortilla pieces.

SECRET INGREDIENT: Young coconuts are green on the outside, and can be found at most Latin and Asian markets. To remove the meat, break the coconut in half and use a regular spoon or ice cream scoop to scrape out the meat. For the best taste, remove as much of the brown skin as possible before adding to the ceviche.

PICADILLO EMPANADAS

MAKES 12 EMPANADAS • PREP TIME: 20 MINUTES • COOK TIME: 55 MINUTES

Empanadas, now a popular snack food throughout Mexico and Latin America, originated in Galicia, Spain—in the northwestern corner of the country right above Portugal. My brother, who lived in that region for many years, always had fresh local empanadas ready to eat whenever I visited. One of my favorite things about Galician empanadas was their super-flaky crust. After picking up some basic baking tips working at Spiral Diner & Bakery in Dallas, I've been able to replicate that perfect empanada crust to accommodate many of my favorite Mexican fillings. These delightfully flaky empanadas, made with vegan butter and cream cheese, are stuffed with one of my absolute favorite fillers, northern Mexican–style picadillo.

FOR THE DOUGH
2 (8-ounce) containers vegan cream cheese
1 cup vegan butter
3½ cups all-purpose flour

FOR THE EMPANADAS
1 tablespoon vegetable oil
½ medium onion, diced small
3 garlic cloves, minced
1 medium russet potato, peeled and diced small
1 or 2 serrano chiles, seeded and minced
½ tablespoon whole cumin seeds
2 cups TVP, rehydrated with 1½ cups hot water, crumbled
1 (15-ounce) can diced tomatoes, not drained
3 tablespoons chopped cilantro
¼ tablespoon apple cider vinegar
1 teaspoon salt
½ teaspoon freshly ground black pepper
Red salsa, for serving

1. **TO MAKE THE DOUGH:** In a large bowl, mix all the ingredients well.

2. Divide the dough into 12 large balls.

3. On a well-floured surface, roll out the balls into round discs. Set aside.

1. **TO MAKE THE EMPANADAS:** Preheat the oven to 375°F.

2. In a large skillet, heat the oil on medium heat. Sauté the onion, garlic, potato, serrano chiles, and cumin seeds for 10 to 15 minutes, or until the potato is evenly browned. Add the rehydrated TVP crumbles and sauté for 3 to 5 more minutes.

3. Add the tomatoes and their juice, cilantro, vinegar, salt, and pepper. Reduce the heat and simmer 5 to 10 minutes, stirring occasionally. Remove from the heat and set aside.

4. Fill each rolled-out dough disc with about 4 tablespoons of filling. Fold the dough over and seal the edges using a little water. Press a fork along the sealed edges to lock in the seal.

5. Bake on a flat baking sheet 25 to 30 minutes, or until golden brown.

6. Let the empanadas sit for 10 minutes before serving. Serve warm with your favorite red salsa, if desired.

COOKING TIP: Leftover empanadas can be quickly reheated in a microwave. Wrap the empanada in a napkin and microwave for 45 to 50 seconds. Let sit for 1 minute before eating.

TLACOYO

SF

GF

MAKES 6 • PREP TIME: 25 MINUTES • COOK TIME: 20 TO 30 MINUTES

Tlacoyo (pronounced tlah-KO-yoh*) is the ultimate Central Mexican street food. You can find tlacoyo—the torpedo-shaped blue corn "Hot Pocket" of ancient Mexico—day or night on nearly every well-trafficked corner in Mexico City. Always filled with piping hot refried black beans and topped with sautéed nopal cactus, they offer a bite full of culture. Like tamales, tlacoyo-making can be a fun activity for friends and family. Party guests at Casa Garza love filling and folding their own torpedoes. The bright blue corn masa is a nostalgic throwback to Play-Doh cooking games from childhood.*

FOR THE BATTER
1½ cups stone-ground blue cornmeal
¼ cup corn masa flour
½ teaspoon salt
1 cup warm water

FOR THE TLACOYO
Nonstick cooking spray
¾ cup Refried Black Beans (page 171)
1 tablespoon canola oil
½ medium white or yellow onion, sliced
1 large nopal cactus pad, dethorned, peeled, and roughly chopped
2 tablespoons chopped cilantro
Salt
⅛ cup Almond Queso Cotija (page 73) (optional)
Red or green salsa, for serving

1. **TO MAKE THE BATTER:** Cut twelve 9-by-12-inch sheets of waxed paper for the tortilla press.

2. In a large bowl, mix together the blue cornmeal, corn masa flour, and salt. Add the water and combine.

3. Divide the masa into six equal portions and form into football-shaped rolls.

4. Line the bottom of the tortilla press with a sheet of waxed paper and place one masa roll in the center of the press. Cover the roll with another piece of waxed paper. Press the masa into a thin disc. Remove the masa disc, still between the waxed paper sheets, and set aside.

5. Repeat until all the rolls have been pressed.

1. **TO MAKE THE TLACOYO:** Preheat an electric griddle to 350°F. If you don't have an electric griddle, you can use a stovetop griddle on medium heat. Lightly spray the griddle with nonstick cooking spray.

2. Peel the top sheet of waxed paper carefully from one disc of pressed masa. Line the center of the disc with 2 tablespoons of Refried Black Beans.

3. Using the bottom sheet of waxed paper and your hands, fold the four corners of the disc over the beans—try not to leave any of the beans exposed. Once the beans are sealed in, use your fingers to shape the soft dough into a torpedo shape (fat in the middle and tapered on the ends), making sure none of the beans squirt out. The dough will be a bit sticky, but use the wax paper to manipulate it. Repeat until all the tlacoyos are formed.

4. Place the tlacoyo directly onto the griddle, folded side down, waxed paper facing up. Peel the waxed paper carefully from the top of the tlacoyo. Cook 7 to 10 minutes on each side, or until browned.

5. While the tlacoyos are cooking, in a large skillet, heat the oil and sauté the onion until translucent. Add the nopal cactus and sauté until tender. Add the cilantro and season with salt. Mix. Remove from the heat and set aside.

6. Top each cooked hot tlacoyo with the nopal and onion sauté, and sprinkle with a teaspoon of Almond Queso Cotija, if using. Serve with a side of red or green salsa of your choice.

SECRET INGREDIENT: Stone-ground blue corn can be found at many natural grocers and online. If you can't find it in your area, use stone-ground white or yellow cornmeal, which you can find at most major supermarkets.

BLACK BEAN TAMALES

MAKES 12 TAMALES • PREP TIME: 15 MINUTES, PLUS 1 HOUR SOAKING TIME •
COOK TIME: 50 MINUTES, PLUS 15 MINUTES RESTING TIME

Tamal-making is a food ritual that has been part of Mexican life since Mesoamerican times. They date as far back as 5,000 BCE and are perhaps the best example of Mexican communal cooking. Preparation is complex and time-consuming, so several people usually make them together. In Grandma's kitchen growing up, making tamales was an all-day event. We made dozens upon dozens to give away as gifts for friends and family around Christmas and New Year's. These fluffy black bean tamales were— and still are—a Garza family favorite.

1 (8-ounce) package dried corn husks

FOR THE BATTER
3 cups corn masa flour
1 teaspoon baking powder
1 teaspoon salt
5 tablespoons vegetable shortening
2¾ cups warm water
1 teaspoon Classic Chile Paste
  (page 194)

FOR THE FILLING
2 tablespoons canola oil
1 small yellow onion, diced
2 medium serrano chiles, finely diced
1 large garlic clove, minced
1 (15-ounce) can black beans, drained
  and rinsed
½ cup chopped cilantro
1 cup water
Salt

1. TO PREPARE THE CORN HUSKS: In a large pot, submerge corn husks in hot water for 1 hour to make them pliable.

2. When the husks are pliable, select 12 of the largest and most flexible. Pat dry the selected husks and separate them. Set aside.

1. TO MAKE THE BATTER: In a large bowl, combine the masa flour, baking powder, and salt. Mix well.

2. Add the vegetable shortening and use your hands to combine it with the dry mix.

3. Add the water and Classic Chile Paste, and mix until the batter is even in color. Set aside.

1. **TO MAKE THE FILLING:** In a large skillet, heat the oil on medium heat. Sauté the onion until it's translucent. Add the serrano chiles and garlic, and sauté until the chiles turn bright green. Add the black beans, cilantro, and water.

2. Reduce the heat to medium-low and simmer for 10 minutes or until about half of the water has evaporated. Mash the beans right in the pot, keeping some whole. Season with salt. Cover the beans and set aside.

1. **TO MAKE THE TAMALES:** Place the husk so the smooth side is facing you. It will be shaped roughly like a triangle.

2. Place about 3 to 4 tablespoons of batter in the center of the corn husk. Using the back of a large spoon, spread the batter evenly across the wide end of the husk. Place about 2½ tablespoons of filling down the center of the batter.

3. Gently roll one of the two long sides of the husk over to surround the filling. Twist the narrow bottom once or twice, or fold it over, to finish forming the tamal. Repeat until all 12 husks are used.

4. In groups of 3 or 4, gently tie the tamales together using kitchen twine.

5. Put about 2 inches of water in a large, deep steaming pot. Add a steamer basket, making sure the water line is below the basket. Place the tamales upright in the basket. To keep the tamales standing in the steamer basket, you can fill any empty space with a heat-resistant cup or mug. Just make sure to leave room for the steam to move between the tamales and around the pot.

6. Cover and steam for about 35 to 40 minutes, adding more water to the pot as needed. Remove from the heat.

7. Let the tamales sit, uncovered, in the pot for about 15 minutes, or until they are firm and pull away from the husk easily.

8. Serve the tamales warm with your favorite red salsa.

SIMPLE SWAP: You can replace the shortening in the batter with 4 tablespoons of olive oil. This will give the tamales a light, silky mouthfeel.

OAXACAN-STYLE MUSHROOM TAMALES

MAKES 12 TAMALES • PREP TIME: 10 MINUTES, PLUS 15 MINUTES STEAMING TIME • COOK TIME: 50 MINUTES, PLUS 15 MINUTES RESTING TIME

In Oaxaca and other tropical regions of southern Mexico, banana leaves are the main choice for wrapping tamales. Banana leaves give the corn masa a subtly sweet flavor, which works wonderfully with the woodsy flavor of white button mushrooms. This recipe calls for olive oil, which adds an extra layer of complexity to these silky smooth Oaxacan-style tamales. Enjoy these with Roasted Tomatillo Salsa (page 201).

1 large package fresh banana leaves

FOR THE BATTER
3 cups corn masa flour
1 teaspoon baking powder
1 teaspoon salt
4 tablespoons olive oil
2¾ cups warm water

FOR THE FILLING
1 tablespoon vegetable oil
½ medium yellow onion, diced
1 large garlic clove, minced
1 pound white button
   mushrooms, sliced
1 teaspoon ground cumin
¼ teaspoon dried thyme
½ teaspoon dried Mexican oregano
½ teaspoon salt

1. TO PREPARE THE BANANA LEAVES: Unfold the banana leaves and cut off the long hard central vein at the end.

2. Cut the leaves into 24 unbroken 12-by-8-inch sheets. Rinse the sheets under running water. Place them in the basket of a steamer and steam them for 15 minutes to make them pliable.

3. While they are steaming, cut 12 additional 12-inch strips from the extra leaves for tying up the tamales.

4. Pat dry the steamed sheets and set aside.

1. TO MAKE THE BATTER: In a large bowl, combine the masa flour, baking powder, and salt. Mix well.

2. Add the olive oil and use your hands to combine it with the dry mix.

3. Add the water and mix well. Set aside.

1. TO MAKE THE FILLING: In a large skillet, heat the oil on medium heat. Sauté the onion until it's translucent.

2. Add the garlic, mushrooms, cumin, thyme, oregano, and salt. Sauté until the mushrooms are cooked through, about 7 minutes.

3. Remove from the heat and set aside.

1. **TO MAKE THE TAMALES:** Place about 3 to 4 tablespoons of batter in the center of a banana leaf sheet. Using the back of a large spoon, spread the batter evenly across the sheet, leaving at least an inch of clear space along the short sides of the sheet. Place about 2½ tablespoons of filling down the center of the batter.

2. Gently fold the leaf over to surround the filling, then make a roll. Fold over the bottom and top ends to seal tamal. Wrap the tamal with another banana leaf sheet and tie shut with a pliable but firm strip of banana leaf. Repeat until all 12 tamales are formed.

3. Put about 2 inches of water in a large, deep steaming pot. Add a steamer basket, making sure the water line is below the basket. Place the tamales upright in the basket. To keep the tamales standing in the steamer basket, you can fill any empty space with a heat-resistant cup or mug. Just make sure to leave room for the steam to move between the tamales and around the pot.

4. Cover and steam for about 35 to 40 minutes, adding more water to the pot as needed. Remove from the heat.

5. Let the tamales sit, uncovered, in the pot for about 15 minutes, or until they are firm and pull away from the husk easily.

6. Serve the tamales warm with your favorite green salsa.

SECRET INGREDIENT: Fresh and frozen banana leaves are usually sold in large packages, and only a small portion of them will be usable for this recipe, because some parts will have holes or will tear too easily. You can find fresh banana leaves in the produce section of most Latin and Asian markets.

GARBANZORIZO, BEAN, and CHEESE TAMALES

MAKES 12 TAMALES • PREP TIME: 10 MINUTES, PLUS 15 MINUTES STEAMING TIME •
COOK TIME: 50 MINUTES, PLUS 15 MINUTES RESTING TIME

Get ready for a taste explosion with these protein-packed Garbanzorizo, bean, and cheese tamales! This flavor combination was a Garza family favorite growing up. In my father's northern Mexican hometown of San Fernando, Tamaulipas, refried pintos are the bean of choice and are often used to bulk up meaty fillers. These ranch-style red tamales are a perfect example of how we stretched meat usage at Casa Garza.

1 (8-ounce) package dried corn husks

FOR THE BATTER
3 cups corn masa flour
1 teaspoon baking powder
1 teaspoon salt
5 tablespoons vegetable shortening
2¾ cups warm water

FOR THE FILLING
2 tablespoons vegetable oil
1 small yellow onion, finely diced
1 cup Garbanzorizo (page 242)
1 cup Spicy Refried Pinto Beans
   (page 174)
1 cup vegan shredded white cheese
Salt

1. TO PREPARE THE CORN HUSKS: In a large pot, submerge corn husks in hot water for 1 hour to make them pliable.

2. When the husks are pliable, select 12 of the largest and most flexible. Pat dry the selected husks and separate them. Set aside.

1. TO MAKE THE BATTER: In a large bowl, combine the masa flour, baking powder, and salt. Mix well.

2. Add the vegetable shortening and use your hands to combine it with the dry mix.

3. Add the water and mix well. Set aside.

1. **TO MAKE THE FILLING:** In a large skillet, heat the oil on medium heat. Sauté the onion until it's translucent.

2. Add the Garbanzorizo, Spicy Refried Pinto Beans, and cheese and stir, adding 1 to 2 tablespoons of water if needed, and cook until heated through.

3. Season with salt and remove from the heat. Set aside.

1. **TO MAKE THE TAMALES:** Place the husk so the smooth side is facing you. It will be shaped roughly like a triangle.

2. Place about 3 to 4 tablespoons of batter in the center of the corn husk. Using the back of a large spoon, spread the batter evenly across the wide end of the husk. Place about 2½ tablespoons of filling down the the center of the batter.

3. Gently roll one of the two long sides of the husk over to surround the filling. Twist the narrow bottom once or twice, or fold it over, to finish forming the tamal. Repeat until all 12 husks are used.

4. In groups of 3 or 4, gently tie the tamales together using kitchen twine.

5. Put about 2 inches of water in a large, deep steaming pot. Add a steamer basket, making sure the water line is below the basket. Place the tamales upright in the basket. To keep the tamales standing in the steamer basket, you can fill any empty space with a heat-resistant cup or mug. Just make sure to leave room for the steam to move between the tamales and around the pot.

6. Cover and steam for about 35 to 40 minutes, adding more water to the pot as needed. Remove from the heat.

7. Let the tamales sit, uncovered, in the pot for about 15 minutes, or until they are firm and pull away from the husk easily.

8. Serve the tamales warm with your favorite red salsa.

COOKING TIP: Leftover tamales can be frozen. To reheat, steam them straight from the freezer for 25 to 30 minutes.

NORTHERN MEXICAN CHICKEN-STYLE SETAS TAMALES

MAKES 12 TAMALES • PREP TIME: 10 MINUTES, PLUS 15 MINUTES STEAMING TIME • COOK TIME: 50 MINUTES, PLUS 15 MINUTES RESTING TIME

Oyster mushrooms are my go-to swap for most chicken recipes. They work exceptionally well in these northern Mexican red tamales. My family in northern Mexico typically use chicken thighs and legs for tamales, reserving the breasts for other dishes. Chopped small and just cooked through, oyster mushrooms do a fantastic job mimicking the taste and texture of tender chicken meat. This recipe also calls for freshly ground cumin seeds, which are sautéed with onion and garlic to bring out their deep, complex flavor.

1 (8-ounce) package dried corn husks

FOR THE BATTER
3 cups corn masa flour
1 teaspoon baking powder
1 teaspoon salt
5 tablespoons vegetable shortening
2¾ cups warm water
1 teaspoon Classic Chile Paste
   (page 194)

FOR THE FILLING
1 tablespoon vegetable oil
½ small yellow onion, finely diced
1 large garlic clove, minced
1 teaspoon whole cumin seeds, ground
   in a molcajete
1 pound oyster mushrooms, chopped
½ teaspoon salt
1 teaspoon Classic Chile Paste
   (page 194)
Red salsa, for serving

1. TO PREPARE THE CORN HUSKS: In a large pot, submerge corn husks in hot water for 1 hour to make them pliable.

2. When the husks are pliable, select 12 of the largest and most flexible. Pat dry the selected husks and separate them. Set aside.

1. TO MAKE THE BATTER: In a large bowl, combine the masa flour, baking powder, and salt. Mix well.

2. Add the vegetable shortening and use your hands to combine it with the dry mix.

3. Add the water and Classic Chile Paste and mix until the batter is even in color. Set aside.

1. **TO MAKE THE FILLING:** In a large skillet, heat the oil on medium heat. Sauté the onion, garlic, and cumin seeds, until the onion is translucent.

2. Add the mushrooms, salt, and Classic Chile Paste and sauté, stirring occasionally, until the mushrooms are cooked through and even in color.

3. Remove from the heat and set aside.

1. **TO MAKE THE TAMALES:** Place the husk so the smooth side is facing you. It will be shaped roughly like a triangle.

2. Place about 3 to 4 tablespoons of batter in the center of the corn husk. Using the back of a large spoon, spread the batter evenly across the wide end of the husk. Place about 2½ tablespoons of filling down the center of the batter.

3. Gently roll one of the two long sides of the husk over to surround the filling. Twist the narrow bottom once or twice, or fold it over, to finish forming the tamal. Repeat until all 12 husks are used.

4. In groups of 3 or 4, gently tie the tamales together using kitchen twine.

5. Put about 2 inches of water in a large, deep steaming pot. Add a steamer basket, making sure the water line is below the basket. Place the tamales upright in the basket. To keep the tamales standing in the steamer basket, you can fill any empty space with a heat-resistant cup or mug. Just make sure to leave room for the steam to move between the tamales and around the pot.

6. Cover and steam for about 35 to 40 minutes, adding more water to the pot as needed. Remove from the heat.

7. Let the tamales sit, uncovered, in the pot for about 15 minutes, or until they are firm and pull away from husk easily.

8. Serve the tamales warm with your favorite red salsa.

COOKING TIP: For a delicious breakfast variation, remove the husks from leftover cold tamales and panfry the tamales with a tablespoon of vegetable oil. Sprinkle with salt and serve hot.

HUITLACOCHE TAMALES

MAKES 12 TAMALES • PREP TIME: 10 MINUTES, PLUS 15 MINUTES STEAMING TIME •
COOK TIME: 1 HOUR, PLUS 15 MINUTES RESTING TIME

Huitlacoche (also spelled cuitlacoche, *but always pronounced*
weet-lah-KO-cheh) *is a Mexican delicacy also known as corn truffle or
corn mushroom. It's a fungus that grows naturally on ears of corn, and is
packed with muscle-building lysine and cholesterol-cutting beta-glucans.
In Mexico, huitlacoche is used to add a smoky flavor to soups, quesadillas,
and other dishes. Each time I visit Mexico City, I stop by a small tamale
restaurant called El Corazón de Tamal in the hip Roma neighborhood to
feast on their delicious huitlacoche tamales. Skip the customs line and
head over to your nearest Latin market to grab a can of huitlacoche so you
can enjoy this wonderful delicacy.*

1 (8-ounce) package dried corn husks

FOR THE BATTER
3 cups corn masa flour
1 teaspoon baking powder
1 teaspoon salt
5 tablespoons vegetable shortening
2¾ cups warm water

FOR THE FILLING
2 tablespoons vegetable oil
1 small yellow onion, diced
1 small poblano chile, diced
½ cup white corn kernels, frozen
   or fresh
1 (7-ounce) can huitlacoche
1 cup fresh epazote leaves, chopped
1 cup water
Salt

1. TO PREPARE THE CORN HUSKS: In a large pot, submerge corn husks in hot water for 1 hour to make them pliable.

2. When the husks are pliable, select 12 of the largest and most flexible. Pat dry the selected husks and separate them. Set aside.

1. TO MAKE THE BATTER: In a large bowl, combine the masa flour, baking powder, and salt. Mix well.

2. Add the vegetable shortening and use your hands to combine it with the dry mix.

3. Add the water and mix well. Set aside.

1. TO MAKE THE FILLING: In a large skillet, heat the oil on medium heat. Sauté the onion until it's translucent. Add the poblano chile, and sauté until the chile is bright green. Add the corn kernels, huitlacoche, epazote, and water.

2. Reduce the heat to medium-low and simmer for 15 to 20 minutes or until the water has nearly evaporated. Season with salt. Set aside.

1. TO MAKE THE TAMALES: Place the husk so the smooth side is facing you. It will be shaped roughly like a triangle.

2. Place about 3 to 4 tablespoons of batter in the center of the corn husk. Using the back of a large spoon, spread the batter evenly across the wide end of the husk. Place about 2½ tablespoons of filling down the center of the batter.

3. Gently roll one of the two long sides of the husk over to surround the filling. Twist the narrow bottom once or twice, or fold it over, to finish forming the tamal. Repeat until all 12 husks are used.

4. In groups of 3 or 4, gently tie the tamales together using kitchen twine.

5. Put about 2 inches of water in a large, deep steaming pot. Add a steamer basket, making sure the water line is below the basket. Place the tamales upright in the basket. To keep the tamales standing in the steamer basket, you can fill any empty space with a heat-resistant cup or mug. Just make sure to leave room for the steam to move between the tamales and around the pot.

6. Cover and steam for about 35 to 40 minutes, adding more water to the pot as needed. Remove from the heat.

7. Let the tamales sit, uncovered, in the pot for about 15 minutes, or until they are firm and pull away from husk easily.

8. Serve the tamales warm with your favorite green salsa.

SECRET INGREDIENT: Huitlacoche has a naturally salty flavor, so go easy on the salt when preparing the filling.

HUITLACOCHE QUESADILLAS

MAKES 12 QUESADILLAS • PREP TIME: 25 MINUTES • COOK TIME: 20 MINUTES

Huitlacoche is finally having its heyday in the fine dining scene. The traditional Mexican delicacy, with its smoky, earthy flavor, is popping up on menus all across the globe. Huitlacoche really shines in this quesadilla recipe, adding a deep complexity to this classic street snack. Sautéed with fresh epazote and sweet white corn, these quesadillas are sure to become a favorite among both your foodie friends and your family.

FOR THE DOUGH
2 cups corn masa flour
½ teaspoon salt
1½ cups warm water

FOR THE QUESADILLAS
1 tablespoon vegetable oil
½ small yellow onion, finely diced (about ½ cup)
4 large epazote leaves, chopped
½ cup white corn kernels, frozen or fresh
1 (7-ounce) can huitlacoche
Nonstick cooking spray
¾ cup vegan shredded white cheese

1. **TO MAKE THE DOUGH:** Cut twenty-four 8-by-12-inch sheets of waxed paper for the tortilla press.

2. In a large bowl, mix together the corn masa flour and salt. Add the water and combine.

3. Divide the masa into 12 equal portions and form into football-shaped rolls.

4. Line the bottom of the tortilla press with a sheet of waxed paper and place one masa roll in the center of the press. Cover the roll with another piece of waxed paper. Press the masa into a thin disc. Remove the masa disc, still between the waxed paper sheets, and set aside.

5. Repeat until all the rolls have been pressed.

1. **TO MAKE THE QUESADILLAS:** Heat the oil in a large skillet on medium-high heat. Add the onion and sauté until translucent. Add the epazote and corn kernels. Sauté the corn until it is slightly toasted, about 3 minutes, stirring occasionally. Add the huitlacoche and sauté for another 1 to 2 minutes, stirring constantly. Remove from the heat and set aside.

2. Heat a large nonstick griddle or skillet on medium heat and lightly spray with nonstick cooking spray. Peel the top sheet of waxed paper carefully from one disc of pressed masa. Place the disc directly onto the griddle, waxed paper facing up. Peel the waxed paper carefully from the top, making sure to not to tear the disc. Spread 1 tablespoon of cheese and about 1½ tablespoons of huitlacoche filling evenly over the masa disc.

3. When the cheese starts to melt, fold the disc in half and cook for about 1 to 1½ minutes. Flip and cook another 1 to 1½ minutes on the other side, or until the cheese is melted and the quesadilla is crispy on both sides. Remove from the heat and repeat with the other quesadillas.

4. Serve quesadillas hot with your favorite green salsa.

SECRET INGREDIENT: This recipe calls for white corn, which is sweeter than the yellow variety. Try out both to see which flavor best suits your taste.

COOKING TIP: Using store-bought tortillas in this recipe is a good option if you're short on time.

SWEET POTATO AND BLACK BEAN EMPANADAS

MAKES 12 EMPANADAS • PREP TIME: 20 MINUTES • COOK TIME: 50 MINUTES, PLUS 10 MINUTES RESTING TIME

Sweet potatoes have been cultivated in Mexico since pre-Hispanic times, and were considered one of the four most important crops to the ancient Maya. The Maya used sweet potatoes to extend maize-based recipes like pozoles and atoles when corn was scarce. Sweet potatoes remain a staple crop in Mexico. In Veracruz, you can find sweet potatoes in various colors, including purple, deep orange, pale orange-yellow, and even white. Paired with protein-packed black beans, this delicious combination makes the perfect sweet and savory empanada.

FOR THE DOUGH

2 (8-ounce) containers vegan cream cheese
1 cup vegan butter
3½ cups all-purpose flour

FOR THE EMPANADAS

2 tablespoons vegetable oil
1 large sweet potato, peeled and diced small
½ medium onion, diced small
3 garlic cloves, minced
1 teaspoon whole cumin seed
1 teaspoon salt
1 teaspoon freshly ground black pepper
2 (15-ounce) cans black beans, drained and rinsed

1. TO MAKE THE DOUGH: In a large bowl, mix all the ingredients well.

2. Divide the dough into 12 large balls.

3. On a well-floured surface, roll out the balls into round discs. Set aside.

1. **TO MAKE THE EMPANADAS:** Preheat the oven to 375°F.

2. In a large skillet, heat the oil on medium heat. Add the sweet potato and cook for 7 minutes, or until it begins to soften. Add the onion, garlic, cumin seeds, salt, and pepper, and continue cooking until the sweet potato begins to brown, about 7 to 10 more minutes. Add the beans and heat through.

3. Fill each rolled-out dough disc with about 4 tablespoons of filling. Fold the dough over and seal the edges using a little water. Press a fork along the sealed edges to lock in the seal.

4. Bake on a flat baking sheet 25 to 30 minutes, or until golden brown.

5. Let the empanadas sit for 10 minutes before serving. Serve warm or cold.

COOKING TIP: Empanada dough rolls better when it's cold. If you have time, let it rest in the refrigerator overnight.

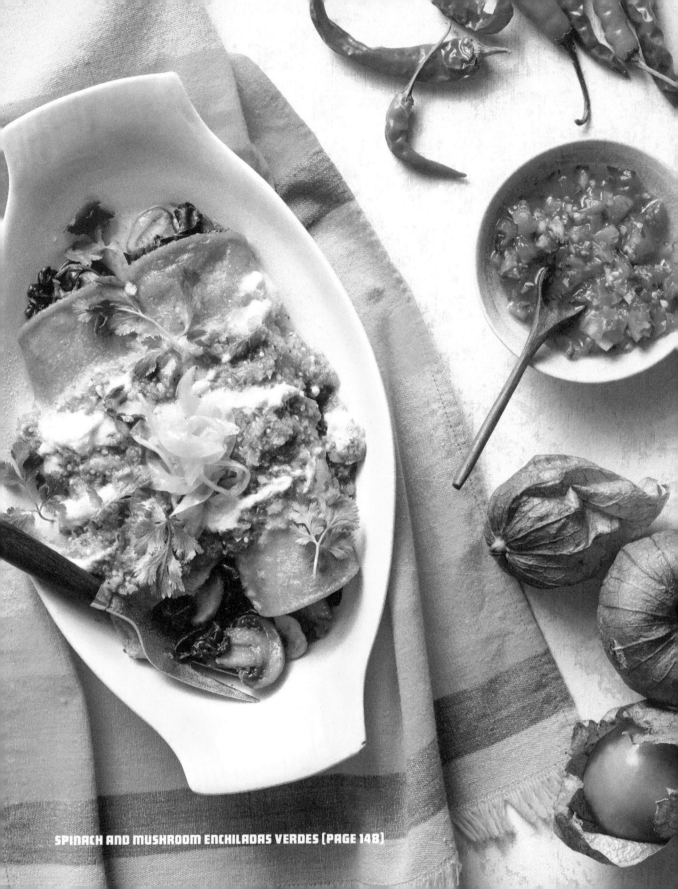

SPINACH AND MUSHROOM ENCHILADAS VERDES [PAGE 148]

Chapter 6

BURRITOS, FAJITAS, AND MÁS

EL ORIGINAL

MAKES 4 BURRITOS • PREP TIME: 15 MINUTES • COOK TIME: 15 MINUTES

Although burritos are largely considered American food by many Mexicans, it's impossible to write a Mexican cookbook without including them. For this plant-based version of the traditional Ciudad Juárez–style burrito, we're stuffing fluffy flour tortillas with the simple yet perfect combo of spicy refried pintos and soy beef-style crumbles.

1 tablespoon olive oil
¼ cup white onion, diced small
2 garlic cloves, minced
1 teaspoon ground cumin
1 teaspoon chili powder
1 teaspoon dried Mexican oregano
1 cup TVP, rehydrated with 2 cups warm water for 15 minutes, crumbled

¼ teaspoon salt
¼ teaspoon freshly ground black pepper
¾ cup Spicy Refried Pinto Beans (page 174)
4 (8-inch) flour tortillas
1 cup Chunky Red Salsa (page 200)

1. Heat the oil in a skillet over medium heat. Sauté the onion and garlic for 4 minutes. Add the cumin, chili powder, and oregano, and stir. Add the TVP and sauté for about 7 minutes, or until nicely browned. Season with salt and pepper and remove from the heat.

2. Reheat the Spicy Refried Pinto Beans in a small saucepan on medium heat (or in the microwave) until warm.

3. Warm the tortillas in a pan, microwave, or grill (my favorite!) until they are pliable.

4. Spread half of the Spicy Refried Pinto Beans on the warm tortilla near the center, then spoon approximately half the TVP mixture into the center of each tortilla.

5. Fold up the bottom half of the tortilla to meet the top half. Hold the bottom edge down and drag it toward you, pulling the filling into the center. Leave the bottom edge folded over the filling. About one-third of the unfilled tortilla should be sticking out the top. Fold both sides in. Your tortilla should now look a bit like an envelope. Roll the filled side up toward the "envelope flap" at the top to seal your burrito. Top with Chunky Red Salsa and serve.

SIMPLE SWAP: For a steak-style version of this classic burrito, try using Mexican Seasoned Seitan (page 239) instead of TVP. Simply dice the seitan and follow the recipe.

BAJA BURRITOS WITH MANGO SALSA

MAKES 2 BURRITOS • PREP TIME: 10 MINUTES • COOK TIME: 15 MINUTES

Seafood-Style Albondigas (meatballs) star in this tropical Baja burrito. It makes the perfect picnic lunch for a day at the beach. Made by combining potatoes, chickpeas, palm hearts, and a touch of dulse flakes to give them a taste of the sea, the albondigas are tightly wrapped in a large flour tortilla with all the classic Baja California fixings—red cabbage, tropical fruit salsas, and spicy chipotle mayo. Enjoy this Baja burrito hot or cold.

6 Seafood-Style Albondigas (page 81)
2 (12-inch) flour tortillas
½ cup shredded red cabbage
½ cup vegan chipotle mayo

½ cup Mango Salsa (page 204)
½ cup Avocado Tomatillo Salsa
   (page 202)

1. If you have the Seafood-Style Albondigas made, reheat them in a nonstick pan with a little nonstick cooking spray until they are warmed through, about 3 minutes each side. If they are not made, start to build the burrito after they are freshly cooked.

2. In a skillet on medium heat, warm the tortillas just until they are pliable.

3. Lay them out and layer the burrito fillings on top: shredded cabbage on one half, mayo on the other, followed by the hot Seafood-Style Albondigas, and finally, the Mango Salsa and Tomatillo Salsa.

4. Fold up the bottom half of the tortilla to meet the top half. Hold the bottom edge down and drag it toward you, pulling the filling into the center. Leave the bottom edge folded over the filling. About one-third of the unfilled tortilla should be sticking out the top. Fold both sides in. Your tortilla should now look a bit like an envelope. Roll the filled side up toward the "envelope flap" at the top to seal your burrito.

COOKING TIP: For toasted burritos, heat a skillet on medium heat, put your burritos in, and press them with another heavy skillet. Toast for about 3 to 4 minutes per side.

BREAKFAST BURRITOS

MAKES 2 BURRITOS • PREP TIME: 10 MINUTES • COOK TIME: 30 MINUTES

Ah, the breakfast burrito. When a tiny little breakfast taquito just won't do, fill up with this big, bad heavyweight breakfast champion. Stuffed with hearty potatoes, tofu huevos, smoky tempeh bacon, avocado, and vegan Cheddar, this hunger fighter will keep you fueled for hours. Enjoy this quick and easy burrito recipe any time of the day.

2 tablespoons olive oil
1 small russet potato, peeled and
     diced small
½ cup tempeh bacon, chopped
½ white onion, diced small
½ teaspoon ground cumin
¼ teaspoon salt
¼ teaspoon freshly ground
     black pepper

2 garlic cloves, minced
1 cup Tofu Huevos (page 237)
½ cup vegan shredded Cheddar cheese
2 (12-inch) flour tortillas
½ medium avocado, peeld and sliced
½ cup Chunky Red Salsa
     (page 200), optional

1. Heat the oil in a skillet over medium heat. Sauté the potatoes 12 minutes, or until they are softened. Add the tempeh bacon, onion, cumin, salt, pepper, and garlic. Sauté 4 more minutes. Fold in the Tofu Huevos and heat through. Stir in the cheese and remove from the heat.

2. In a skillet on medium heat, warm the tortillas just until they are pliable. Spoon about half the filling into the center of each tortilla and top with half the avocado slices.

3. Fold up the bottom half of the tortilla to meet the top half. Hold the bottom edge down and drag it toward you, pulling the filling into the center. Leave the bottom edge folded over the filling. About one-third of the unfilled tortilla should be sticking out the top. Fold both sides in. Your tortilla should now look a bit like an envelope. Roll the filled side up toward the "envelope flap" at the top to seal your burrito.

4. Top with warm Chunky Red Salsa, if you'd like, or wrap it up to go in aluminum foil.

SIMPLE SWAP: Swap any kind of plant-based breakfast meat for the tempeh bacon. I like to use Garbanzorizo (page 242) for variety.

JACKFRUIT CARNITAS BURRITOS

MAKES 2 BURRITOS • PREP TIME: 10 MINUTES • COOK TIME: 30 MINUTES

This burrito has "hip factor" written all over it. Before your eyes roll, carnitas ("little meats") have been around for a while. The dish originally comes from the Mexican state of Michoacán and has seen a spike in popularity in the US. Jackfruit has also been around for a long time and is also experiencing a spike in popularity in Latin America and North America, due to its ability to mimic the textures of pulled pork and carnitas. Here we take the seasonings of traditional carnitas and marry them to the texture of jackfruit for a healthy update to an evolving classic.

1 tablespoon olive oil
¾ cup jackfruit carnitas, prepared
    as for Jackfruit Carnitas
    Tortas (page 99)
½ cup frozen corn kernels, thawed
3 tablespoons Roasted Tomatillo Salsa
    (page 201), plus 1 cup to serve
½ cup cooked or canned black beans,
    drained and rinsed

½ cup Cilantro Lime Rice (page 162)
¼ teaspoon salt
¼ teaspoon freshly ground
    black pepper
½ cup vegan shredded white cheese
2 (12-inch) flour tortillas
1 avocado, peeled and sliced

1. Heat the oil in a large skillet over medium heat. Sauté the jackfruit carnitas 5 minutes, or until hot. Add the corn, sauté for 4 minutes, add in Roasted Tomatillo Salsa. Fold in the beans and Cilantro Lime Rice, and sprinkle with the salt and pepper. Heat through. Stir in the cheese and remove from the heat.

2. Warm the tortillas in a pan, microwave, or grill (my favorite!) until they are pliable.

3. Spoon about half the filling into the center of each tortilla. Arrange half the sliced avocado on top of each.

4. Fold up the bottom half of the tortilla to meet the top half. Hold the bottom edge down and drag it toward you,

pulling the filling into the center. Leave the bottom edge folded over the filling. About one-third of the unfilled tortilla should be sticking out the top. Fold both sides in. Your tortilla should now look a bit like an envelope. Roll the filled side up toward the "envelope flap" at the top to seal your burrito.

5. Top each burrito with ½ cup of warm Roasted Tomatillo Salsa.

SECRET INGREDIENT: When cooking jackfruit, to achieve the best texture, make sure to cook much of the water out of the fruit. One of the ways to do this is to first roast the jackfruit for 15 to 20 minutes at 400°F.

BURRITOS ENMOLADOS

MAKES 2 BURRITOS • PREP TIME: 10 MINUTES • COOK TIME: 30 MINUTES

Pull out the knife and fork—and perhaps a few extra napkins—for this saucy twist on the original handheld burrito. Enmolado means "drenched in mole sauce." For these enmolados, I fill large flour tortillas with Mexican black beans, sweet potatoes, and poblano chiles, then drown them in my savory chocolate Brown Mole, and a drizzle of Cashew Crema Mexicana to balance out the rich, bold flavors. Enjoy this dish on a day of indulgence.

2 tablespoons olive oil
1 small sweet potato, peeled and diced
½ white onion, diced small
½ poblano chile, diced small
½ teaspoon ground cumin
½ teaspoon chili powder
½ teaspoon dried Mexican oregano
¼ teaspoon salt

¼ teaspoon freshly ground
  black pepper
2 garlic cloves, minced
1 cup Brown Mole (page 196), divided
1 (15.5-ounce) can black beans, drained
  and rinsed
2 (12-inch) flour tortillas
½ cup red onion, diced small
Cashew Crema Mexicana (page 230)

1. Heat the oil in a skillet over medium heat. Sauté the sweet potato 10 minutes, or until softened. Add the onion, poblano chile, cumin, chili powder, oregano, salt, pepper, and garlic. Sauté 4 more minutes. Add ½ cup of the Brown Mole sauce and the black beans, and heat through.

2. Heat the tortillas in a pan, microwave, or grill until they are pliable. Spoon about half the filling into the center of each tortilla.

3. Fold up the bottom half of the tortilla to meet the top half. Hold the bottom edge down and drag it toward you, pulling the filling into the center. Leave the bottom edge folded over the filling.

About one-third of the unfilled tortilla should be sticking out the top. Fold both sides in. Your tortilla should now look a bit like an envelope. Roll the filled side up toward the "envelope flap" at the top to seal your burrito.

4. Top each with ¼ cup Brown Mole. Sprinkle with red onions and drizzle with Cashew Crema Mexicana.

COOKING TIP: This is a very rich, heavy dish, and flour tortillas don't hold together too well after being drenched in a sauce like this. If you don't think you can eat the whole thing in one sitting, cut the burrito in half before pouring on the mole and save the other half for later.

BLACK BEAN, RICE, and PLANTAIN BURRITOS

MAKES 2 BURRITOS • PREP TIME: 15 MINUTES • COOK TIME: 15 MINUTES

This burrito takes a little of this and a little of that and something from over there. It might seem like a hodgepodge, but the balance of flavors is a classic in the burrito world. The earthiness and heartiness of the black bean—the very first type of bean to be domesticated—meets its match in the soft and sweet sautéed plantain.

1 tablespoon olive oil
¼ cup white onion, diced small
1 jalapeño chile, seeded and
    diced small
1 large ripe plantain, peeled and sliced
1 teaspoon ground cumin
1 teaspoon dried Mexican oregano
2 garlic cloves, minced
1 (15-ounce) can black beans, drained
    and rinsed

¼ teaspoon salt
¼ teaspoon freshly ground
    black pepper
¾ cup Arroz Rojo (page 163)
2 (12-inch) flour tortillas
¾ cup vegan shredded white cheese
1 whole avocado, peeled and sliced
3 tablespoons chopped cilantro

1. Heat the oil in a skillet over medium heat. Sauté the onion, jalapeño, and plantain for 8 minutes. Add the cumin and oregano and stir. Add the garlic and beans and sauté for about 3 minutes or until the beans are warm. Sprinkle with the salt and pepper.

2. Stir in the Arroz Rojo and heat through.

3. Heat the tortillas in a pan, microwave, or grill until they are pliable.

4. Spoon about half the beans and Arroz Rojo filling into the center of each tortilla. Top with half the cheese, sliced avocados, and cilantro.

5. Fold up the bottom half of the tortilla to meet the top half. Hold the bottom edge down and drag it toward you, pulling the filling into the center. Leave the bottom edge folded over the filling. About one-third of the unfilled tortilla should be sticking out the top. Fold both sides in. Your tortilla should now look a bit like an envelope. Roll the filled side up toward the "envelope flap" at the top to seal your burrito.

SIMPLE SWAP: If you would like to try a different grain instead of rice, try quinoa or the very versatile and easy to prepare amaranth. Season either one with salt, pepper, and a squeeze of lime. Give them a try!

CLASSIC BEEF-STYLE FAJITAS

MAKES 8 TO 10 FAJITAS • PREP TIME: 20 MINUTES, PLUS 20 MINUTES
MARINATING TIME • COOK TIME: 20 MINUTES

Believe it or not, the much-adored fajita has been on the food scene for less than a century. While the dish is more Tex-Mex than it is Mexican cuisine, it was Mexican ranch workers living in Texas along the border who invented the now-popular sizzling dish back in the 1930s. The original fajita was made from beef, and the name referred to the actual cut of beef—the skirt steak. Fajitas nowadays are made with a variety of ingredients. This version features pan-seared seitan steak flavored in a spiced beer marinade (I like Negra Modelo or Bohemia beer). Serve this border town classic with Arroz Rojo (page 163) and a side of Spicy Refried Pinto Beans (page 174).

FOR THE MARINADE
½ teaspoon onion powder
½ teaspoon chipotle powder
1 teaspoon garlic powder
1 teaspoon ground cumin
2 teaspoons freshly ground
    black pepper
2 teaspoons salt
2 tablespoons vegetable oil
2 tablespoons dark Mexican beer

FOR THE FAJITAS
1 pound Mexican Seasoned Seitan
    (page 239), cut into
    ½-inch-thick steaks
2 teaspoons vegetable oil
1 tablespoon vegan butter
½ white onion, julienned
½ green bell pepper, julienned
½ red bell pepper, julienned
2 jalapeño chiles, halved lengthwise
½ teaspoon salt
½ teaspoon freshly ground
    black pepper
8 to 10 corn or 6-inch flour tortillas

GARNISH OPTIONS
Pico de Gallo (page 198)
2 limes, quartered
Classic Guacamole (page 235)
Hot sauce

1. **TO MAKE THE MARINADE:** Mix everything except the oil and beer together in a large bowl.

2. Add the oil and beer, and whisk.

1. **TO MAKE THE FAJITAS:** Generously rub the Mexican Seasoned Seitan steaks with the marinade. Marinate for 20 minutes in the refrigerator. Discard the marinade.

2. Heat the oil in a large skillet over medium-high heat. Sear the Mexican Seasoned Seitan about 4 to 5 minutes each side, until nicely browned. Remove from the pan and set aside.

3. In the same pan, melt the butter and sauté the onion, bell pepper, and jalapeños for 5 to 7 minutes. Season with salt and pepper. Remove from the heat.

4. Slice the Mexican Seasoned Seitan into strips. Plate on a large platter with the onion and pepper.

5. Top with the garnishes of your choice.

6. Serve with warm corn tortillas.

COOKING TIP: Make sure there's plenty of ventilation when sautéing jalapeños, as the aromas can get pretty intense.

PORTABELLO FAJITAS

MAKES 8 TO 10 FAJITAS • PREP TIME: 5 MINUTES, PLUS 20 MINUTES MARINATING TIME • COOK TIME: 20 MINUTES

Often served on a sizzling platter with warm tortillas and plenty of condiments, the star of this fajita dish is the meaty portobello mushroom. Throw this large spiced beer-marinated cap on the grill (I like Negra Modelo or Bohemia beer for this dish), and enjoy this modern-day vegan classic with a big bowl of Borracho Beans with Green Chiles (page 175).

FOR THE MARINADE
½ teaspoon onion powder
½ teaspoon chipotle powder
1 teaspoon garlic powder
1 teaspoon ground cumin
2 teaspoons freshly ground
   black pepper
2 teaspoons salt
2 tablespoons vegetable oil
2 tablespoons dark Mexican beer

FOR THE FAJITAS
1 pound portobello mushrooms, stems
   and gills removed
1 tablespoon vegan butter

½ white onion, julienned
½ green bell pepper, julienned
½ red bell pepper, julienned
2 jalapeño chiles, halved lengthwise
½ teaspoon salt
½ teaspoon freshly ground
   black pepper
8 to 10 corn tortillas

GARNISH OPTIONS
1 cup Pico de Gallo (page 198)
2 limes, quartered
1 cup Classic Guacamole (page 235)
Vinegar hot sauce

1. TO MAKE THE MARINADE: Mix everything except the oil and beer together in a large bowl.

2. Add the oil and beer and whisk.

1. TO MAKE THE FAJITAS: Generously rub the mushrooms with the marinade. Marinate for 20 minutes in the refrigerator. Discard the marinade.

2. Grill the mushrooms about 4 to 5 minutes each side over the high heat of a direct flame, or in a hot cast-iron skillet.

3. In large skillet, melt the butter and sauté the onion, bell peppers, and jalapeños for 5 to 7 minutes. Sprinkle

with the salt and pepper. Remove from the heat.

4. Slice the mushrooms into ½-inch strips. Plate on a large platter with the onion and peppers.

5. Top with the garnishes of your choice.

6. Serve with warm corn tortillas.

COOKING TIP: If you don't have a grill, you can cook the mushrooms on the stovetop. Slice them first, then warm 2 tablespoons of vegetable oil in a large skillet over medium-high heat. Sauté the mushrooms for 4 to 5 minutes. Remove from the pan and set aside. Continue to step 3.

PALM HEART SEAFOOD-STYLE FAJITAS

MAKES 8 TO 10 FAJITAS • PREP TIME: 20 MINUTES, PLUS 15 MINUTES SOAKING TIME • COOK TIME: 15 MINUTES

The multitextured layers of hearts of palm make them the perfect substitute for fish, crab, scallops, and calamari in this vegan version of seafood fajitas. Cut on a bias, palm hearts take on the texture of fish and crab. Salad cut, they resemble bits of scallops and calamari. Sautéed with finely julienned onion, mild guajillo chiles, and garlic, these light yet satisfying fajitas are a great way to close out a fun day at the beach—especially for the sea animals!

2 teaspoons vegetable oil
½ white onion, finely julienned
4 guajillo chiles, rehydrated in hot water for 14 minutes, seeded, stemmed, and chopped
4 garlic cloves, minced
1 teaspoon ground cumin
½ teaspoon freshly ground black pepper
1 (14-ounce) can whole hearts of palm, drained, cut on a thin bias

1 tablespoon minced cilantro
8 to 10 corn tortillas

GARNISH OPTIONS
Pico de Gallo (page 198)
2 limes, quartered
Classic Guacamole (page 235)
Vinegar hot sauce

1. Heat the oil in a large skillet over medium-high heat. Sauté the onion for 4 minutes. Add the guajillo chiles and garlic, and sauté another 4 minutes.

2. Add the cumin, pepper, and hearts of palm. Sauté 5 minutes more, until the hearts of palm are browned.

3. Remove from the heat. Fold in the cilantro.

4. Plate on large platter and top with the garnishes of your choice.

5. Serve with warm corn tortillas.

HEAT INDEX: Guajillo chiles are used for this recipe because they add a beautiful red hue to the dish without adding too much heat. For more spice, add one or two chiles de árbol to the mix.

CHICKEN-STYLE OYSTER MUSHROOM FAJITAS

MAKES 8 TO 10 FAJITAS • PREP TIME: 3 MINUTES, PLUS 20 MINUTES
MARINATING TIME • COOK TIME: 20 MINUTES

Though far removed from the original skirt steak fajita, there's no denying the popularity of modern renditions of the now Tex-Mex classic. Among the most popular styles is the chicken fajita, which can easily be made in a multitude of vegan versions available at your neighborhood grocery store. Of course, I almost always use oyster mushrooms to replace chicken because of their remarkable versatility and ability to absorb flavors. And they work incredibly well in this grilled Tex-Mex favorite. The trick is to grill the mushrooms on a direct flame on high heat to really bring out that smoky flavor we all love in fajitas.

FOR THE MARINADE
½ teaspoon onion powder
½ teaspoon chipotle powder
1 teaspoon garlic powder
1 teaspoon ground cumin
2 teaspoons freshly ground
   black pepper
2 teaspoons salt
2 tablespoons vegetable oil
2 tablespoons dark Mexican beer

FOR THE FAJITAS
1½ pounds oyster mushrooms
1 tablespoon vegan butter
½ white onion, julienned
½ green bell pepper, julienned
½ red bell pepper, julienned
2 jalapeño chiles, halved lengthwise
½ teaspoon salt
½ teaspoon freshly ground
   black pepper
8 to 10 corn tortillas

GARNISH OPTIONS
Pico de Gallo (page 198)
2 limes, quartered
Classic Guacamole (page 235)
Hot sauce

1. **TO MAKE THE MARINADE:** Mix everything except the oil and beer together in a large bowl.

2. Add the oil and beer and whisk.

1. **TO MAKE THE FAJITAS:** Generously rub the mushrooms with the marinade. Marinate for 20 minutes in the refrigerator. Discard the marinade.

2. Grill the mushrooms about 4 to 5 minutes each side over the high heat of a direct flame or on a hot cast-iron skillet.

3. In large skillet, melt the butter and sauté the onion, bell peppers, and jalapeños for 5 to 7 minutes. Mix with the salt and pepper. Remove from the heat.

4. Slice the mushrooms into ½-inch strips. Plate on a large platter with the onion and peppers, and the tortillas.

5. Top with the garnishes of your choice.

COOKING TIP: If you don't have a grill, you can cook the mushrooms on the stovetop. Slice them first, then warm 2 tablespoons of vegetable oil in a large skillet over medium-high heat. Sauté the mushrooms for 4 to 5 minutes. Remove the pan and set aside. Continue to step 3.

BEEF-STYLE CHIMICHANGAS

MAKES 2 CHIMICHANGAS • PREP TIME: 15 MINUTES • COOK TIME: 20 MINUTES

There are many stories of who invented the chimichanga, but some say it all began at a restaurant in Arizona when the owner dropped a burrito into hot oil. When she saw what happened, the first thing she said was "Chimichanga!" No matter who created this mouthwatering dish, we're grateful for the fried burrito that fuses the best of two worlds—American comfort food and Mexican eclectic fixings. For this recipe, we combine textured soy crumbles, refried beans, and vegan Cheddar for an amazing dish.

1 tablespoon olive oil
½ white onion, sliced very thin
1 jalapeño chile, seed and cut into thin slices
½ red bell pepper, seeded and cut into thin slices
2 garlic cloves, minced
1 teaspoon ground cumin
1 teaspoon chili powder
1 teaspoon dried Mexican oregano
1 cup TVP, rehydrated with 2 cups warm water for 15 minutes, crumbled

¼ teaspoon salt
¼ teaspoon freshly ground black pepper
¾ cup Spicy Refried Pinto Beans (page 174) or canned refried pinto beans
2 (12-inch) flour tortillas
½ cup vegan shredded Cheddar cheese
2 cups vegetable oil, for frying
½ cup Salsa Ranchera (page 199), warmed
½ cup Pico de Gallo (page 198)

1. Heat the olive oil in a skillet over medium heat. Sauté the onion, jalapeño, bell pepper, and garlic for 4 minutes. Add the cumin, chili powder, oregano, and TVP, and sauté for about 7 minutes or until nicely browned. Season with salt and pepper and remove from the heat.

2. Reheat the refried beans in a small saucepan on medium heat (or in the microwave) until warm.

3. Warm the tortillas until they are pliable.

4. Spread about half the Spicy Refried Pinto Beans on a warm tortilla near the center, sprinkle with cheese, then spoon about half the TVP mixture into the center of each tortilla.

5. Fold up the bottom half of the tortilla to meet the top half. Hold the bottom edge down and drag it toward you, pulling the filling into the center. Leave the bottom edge folded over the filling.

About one-third of the unfilled tortilla should be sticking out the top. Fold both sides in. Your tortilla should now look a bit like an envelope. Roll the filled side up toward the "envelope flap" at the top to seal your chimichanga.

6. Heat the vegetable oil in a deep frying pan on medium-high heat. When the oil is hot, carefully lay the chimichanga in the pan and fry each side for about 5 minutes, or until the entire tortilla is browned. Remove from the pan with tongs or a slotted spoon and let drain or a rack or on a paper towel–lined plate. Repeat with the other chimichanga.

7. Serve with warm Salsa Ranchera and Pico de Gallo.

COOKING TIP: If frying just isn't your thing, feel free to use this filling to build a pan-toasted beef-style burrito.

MASHED POTATO AND POBLANO FLAUTAS

MAKES 12 FLAUTAS • PREP TIME: 10 MINUTES • COOK TIME: 30 MINUTES

Flautas, also known as "tacos dorados" (golden tacos) in Mexico and "taquitos" in some parts of the US, were one of the first Mexican meals mass-produced as flash-frozen foods here in the States. In Mexico, these small flutes are rolled around an assortment of fresh ingredients and deep fried to a golden crisp. For this healthier recipe, I combine mashed potatoes and sautéed poblanos, and bake the flautas to crunchy-on-the-outside, creamy-on-the-inside bliss.

Nonstick cooking spray
1 teaspoon vegetable oil
½ white onion, diced small
1 poblano chile, diced small
1 teaspoon whole cumin seeds
1 teaspoon salt

½ teaspoon freshly ground
   black pepper
3 garlic cloves, minced
2 russet potatoes, baked or
   microwaved, skins discarded
1 tablespoon unsweetened almond milk
12 corn tortillas

1. Preheat the oven to 425°F. Lightly spray a nonstick baking sheet with nonstick cooking spray.

2. Heat the oil in a large skillet over medium-high heat. Sauté the onion and poblano chile for 4 to 5 minutes, or until the onion is translucent. Add the cumin seeds, salt, pepper, and garlic. Sauté 4 more minutes. Remove from the heat.

3. In a large bowl, mix together the onion mixture, cooked potato, and almond milk. Mash well. Some visible chunks are fine.

4. Warm the tortillas until they are pliable.

5. To assemble the flautas, place 2 tablespoons of potato filling in each tortilla and roll it up tightly. Place on the prepared baking sheet. Repeat until all the tortillas are rolled up.

6. Lightly spray the flautas with nonstick cooking spray and place in the oven. Bake 10 to 12 minutes, or until the edges of the tortillas are brown and crispy. Turn the pan around halfway through the cooking time for even cooking.

ORIGIN STORY: In Mexico, rolling up fillings into tortillas is a culinary tradition dating back to the Maya. Flautas, which means "flutes," are a great example of this style of food. They can be either baked or fried to achieve a crispy shell.

BEEF-STYLE FLAUTAS

MAKES 12 FLAUTAS • PREP TIME: 10 MINUTES • COOK TIME: 20 MINUTES

In keeping with the Maya roots of this dish, we will go with baking plant-based beef–filled corn tortillas as opposed to frying, which is a cooking method that didn't exist in Mexico until the Spanish conquistadors arrived. Once you're finished making these, you will love dipping them into your favorite salsa!

Nonstick cooking spray
1 teaspoon vegetable oil
½ white onion, diced small
1 teaspoon whole cumin seeds
1 teaspoon salt
½ teaspoon freshly ground
   black pepper

3 garlic cloves, minced
2 whole chipotle chiles, minced
4 cups TVP, rehydrated with
   3 cups warm water for
   10 minutes, crumbled
1 cup vegan shredded Cheddar cheese
12 corn tortillas

1. Preheat the oven to 425°F. Lightly spray a nonstick baking sheet with nonstick cooking spray.

2. Heat the oil in a large skillet over medium-high heat. Sauté the onion for 4 to 5 minutes, or until it is translucent.

3. Add the cumin seeds, salt, pepper, garlic, chipotles, and TVP. Sauté 5 to 7 more minutes or until browned. Fold in the cheese. Remove from the heat.

4. Warm the tortillas until they are pliable.

5. To assemble the flautas, place 2 tablespoons of TVP filling in each tortilla and roll it up tightly. Place on the prepared baking sheet. Repeat until all the tortillas are rolled up.

6. Lightly spray the flautas with nonstick cooking spray and place in the oven. Bake 10 to 12 minutes, or until the edges of the tortillas are brown and crispy. You may want to flip the flautas halfway through, for an even bake.

7. Serve with your favorite salsa.

COOKING TIP: For the more indulgent fried version, heat ¼ inch to ½ inch of oil in a large frying pan on medium-high heat. Place the flautas seam-side down on the pan and fry for 2 minutes. Flip and fry for another 2 to 3 minutes. Remove from the oil and set aside to cool on a rack before serving.

CLASSIC CHILE RELLENOS

MAKES 2 CHILES • PREP TIME: 35 MINUTES • COOK TIME: 45 MINUTES

Aquafaba—the brine from canned chickpeas—is the unlikely star of this vegan version of Classic Chile Rellenos. The popular dish originated in the East-Central Mexican city of Puebla and is traditionally prepared by charring and peeling poblano chiles, stuffing them with meat, then dipping them in an egg-based batter and deep frying. This take on the relleno is filled with a cheesy soy-beef stuffing, then fried to perfection in an aquafaba-based batter.

FOR THE BATTER
Brine from 2 (15-ounce) cans chickpeas
½ cup all-purpose flour
¼ teaspoon salt
¼ teaspoon freshly ground
   black pepper

FOR THE CHILES
2 large poblano chiles
1 teaspoon olive oil
1 teaspoon vegetable oil
¼ cup white onion, diced small
2 teaspoons ground cumin
1 teaspoon dried Mexican oregano
1 teaspoon salt

½ teaspoon freshly ground
   black pepper
3 garlic cloves, minced
2 cups TVP, rehydrated with 1½ cups
   warm water for 10 minutes, crumbled
⅓ cup vegan shredded Cheddar cheese,
   plus 2 tablespoons for garnish
2 tablespoons vegan cream cheese
2 cups vegetable oil, for frying
2 tablespoons all-purpose flour
¾ cup Salsa Ranchera (page 199)
2 tablespoons Cashew Crema Mexicana
   (page 230)
2 tablespoons cilantro leaves

1. TO MAKE THE BATTER: Drain the chickpea brine into a large mixing bowl.

2. Whisk for at least 5 to 7 minutes. It will begin to turn white and form light peaks as you whisk.

3. When the peaks start to firm up, sift in the flour and whisk until smooth. Sprinkle with the salt and pepper.

1. TO MAKE THE CHILES: Preheat the oven to 425°F.

2. Lightly oil the poblanos with olive oil, and place them on a small pan. Roast for about 10 minutes, turning them halfway through the cooking time. When all sides of the chiles are blistered, remove the chiles from the oven and place them in a bowl. Cover with plastic wrap. Set aside to let the chiles rest so the skin will be easy to remove.

3. Heat the vegetable oil in a large skillet on medium-high heat. Sauté the onion for 4 to 5 minutes, until it is translucent. Add the cumin, oregano, salt, pepper, garlic, and TVP. Sauté for 5 to 7 minutes or until browned. Fold in the cheeses. Remove from the heat.

4. Remove the chiles from the bowl. Using the back side of your knife, gently remove the skin from the chiles. Cut a slit from near the stem going down toward the bottom of the chile, being careful not to cut the chile in half. (You need it intact for stuffing.)

5. Heat 2 cups of oil in a deep skillet on medium-high heat. Divide the TVP mixture in half, and carefully spoon half into one of the chiles.

6. Roll the stuffed chile in the dry flour, then in the batter, being careful to keep all the filling inside the chile. (You can use 2 to 3 wooden toothpicks or a skewer to keep the chile closed.)

7. Place the chile in the hot oil and fry for about 4 to 5 minutes each side or until golden brown.

8. Repeat with the second chile. Let the chiles drain on a wire rack or a paper towel–lined plate.

9. To serve, cover with warm Salsa Ranchera and garnish with Cashew Crema Mexicana, 2 tablespoons cheese, and cilantro.

COOKING TIP: For best results, use a balloon whisk when working with aquafaba. Once your aquafaba has nice firm peaks, sift in the flour and keep whisking until the batter is thick enough to cling to your chile. This is not an easy task and it will take a little time, but be patient and it will happen. The batter should be about the consistency of pancake batter, only fluffier.

ROASTED CHILE RELLENOS

MAKES 2 CHILES • PREP TIME: 20 MINUTES • COOK TIME: 40 MINUTES

Like so many Mexican classic dishes, Chile Rellenos can be prepared in a number of ways. While frying the chiles is absolutely delicious, roasting develops and combines the flavors in a way that only this method can achieve.

Nonstick cooking spray
2 large poblano chiles
1 teaspoon olive oil
1 teaspoon vegetable oil
1 medium sweet potato, peeled and diced small
¼ cup white onion, diced small
1 teaspoon ground cumin
½ teaspoon dried Mexican oregano
1 teaspoon salt

½ teaspoon freshly ground black pepper
2 garlic cloves, minced
½ cup frozen corn kernels, thawed
⅓ cup vegan shredded Cheddar cheese, plus 2 tablespoons for garnish
¾ cup Salsa Ranchera (page 199), plus 4 tablespoons for filling
1 (15-ounce) can black beans, drained and rinsed
2 tablespoons chopped cilantro

1. Preheat the oven to 425°F. Spray a roasting pan with nonstick cooking spray.

2. Lightly oil the poblanos with olive oil, and place them on a small pan. Roast about 10 minutes, turning them halfway through the cooking time. When all sides of the chiles are blistered, remove the chiles from the oven and place them in a bowl. Cover with plastic wrap. Set aside to let the chiles rest so the skin will be easy to remove.

3. Reduce the oven temperature to 400°F.

4. In a skillet, heat the vegetable oil on medium heat. Sauté the sweet potato for about 10 minutes, stirring frequently so it doesn't burn.

5. Add the onion and cook for 4 minutes or until it is translucent. Add the cumin, oregano, salt, pepper, garlic, and corn. Sauté for 3 minutes.

6. Fold in the cheese, 4 tablespoons of Salsa Ranchera, and the beans and heat through. Remove from the heat.

7. Remove the chiles from the bowl. Using the back side of your knife, gently remove the skin from the chiles. Cut a slit from near the stem going down toward the bottom of the chile, being careful not to cut the chile in half. (You need it intact for stuffing.)

8. Divide the filling into two portions and gently fill each chile with half the mixture. Place the stuffed chiles onto the prepared roasting pan and roast for 10 to 12 minutes, or until the filling is browned and bubbling.

9. Remove from the oven and let the rellenos rest.

10. Plate and cover with warm Salsa Ranchera. Garnish each chile with 1 tablespoon cheese and 1 tablespoon cilantro.

COOKING TIP: If you have access to an open flame, you can char the chiles faster. The end result is essentially the same.

CHILES en NOGADA

MAKES 2 CHILES • PREP TIME: 30 MINUTES • COOK TIME: 25 MINUTES

Chiles en Nogada are a prime example of combining the strengths of a range of whole foods into one beautifully balanced dish. The mild tang and spice of poblano chiles meet their counterparts in the sweet and savory fillings of fruit and nuts. And, not only is this dish balanced with flavors, but once the chile is filled, you will have built a meal that displays the three colors of the Mexican flag: green from the chile, white from the sauce, and red from the fruit. Hopefully, you are as proud of sharing this dish with friends and family as the people of Puebla are for sharing it with the world!

FOR THE SAUCE

¼ cup Cashew Crema Mexicana (page 230)
½ cup walnuts, rinsed and peeled of as much dark skin as possible
½ cup white bread, crust removed and cut into small cubes
1 cup unsweetened almond or rice milk
¼ teaspoon salt
¼ teaspoon white pepper

FOR THE CHILES

Nonstick cooking spray
2 large poblano chiles
1 teaspoon olive oil
1 teaspoon vegetable oil
1½ cups Picadillo from Picadillo Empanada recipe (page 104)
⅓ cup raisins
¼ cup walnuts, chopped finely
½ cup pomegranate seeds
½ cup finely chopped flat leaf parsley
⅓ cup Almond Queso Cotija (page 73)

1. TO MAKE THE SAUCE: In a large blender, add Cashew Crema Mexicana, walnuts, bread, almond or rice milk, salt, and pepper, and purée until very smooth.

2. Set aside.

1. TO MAKE THE CHILES: Preheat the oven to 425°F. Spray a roasting pan with nonstick cooking spray.

2. Lightly oil the poblanos with olive oil, and place them on a small pan. Roast about 10 minutes, turning them halfway through the cooking time. When all sides of the chiles are blistered, remove the chiles from the oven and place them in a bowl. Cover with plastic wrap. Set aside to let the chiles rest so the skin will be easy to remove.

3. Reduce the oven temperature to 400°F.

4. In a skillet, heat 1 teaspoon of vegetable oil on medium heat. Sauté the Picadillo for about 5 to 7 minutes, stirring frequently.

5. Add the raisins and chopped walnuts and heat through. Remove the mixture from the heat.

6. Remove the chiles from the bowl. Using the back side of your knife, gently remove the skin from the chiles. This can also be done with your hands. Cut a slit from near the stem going down toward the bottom of the chile, being careful not to cut the chile in half. (You need it intact for stuffing.)

7. Divide the Picadillo mixture into two portions and gently fill each chile with half the mixture. Place the stuffed chiles onto the prepared roasting pan and roast for 10 to 12 minutes, or until the filling is browned and bubbling.

8. Remove the chiles from the oven and let them rest for 3 minutes.

9. Transfer the chiles to serving plates and coat with nogada sauce. Garnish the stem end of the chile with pomegranate seeds and the bottom end of the chile with parsley. Top with Almond Queso Cotija.

COOKING TIP: Nogada sauce can be made a day ahead, which will help it develop more complexity. Simply refrigerate after making the sauce, then warm up slightly and stir before serving.

SPINACH and MUSHROOM ENCHILADAS VERDES

MAKES 8 ENCHILADAS • PREP TIME: 20 MINUTES • COOK TIME: 30 MINUTES

The enchilada is an ancient dish that has gone through many changes since its pre-Hispanic origins. The now vastly transformed enchilada is a popular comfort food enjoyed throughout the world. One key difference is the amount of salsa we use. In ancient times, filled tortilla flutes were dipped in chile sauce; now they're drenched in sauce. (I say that's a good thing!) This modern take on the Aztec classic, featuring Roasted Tomatillo Salsa, fresh spinach, white button mushrooms, and Cashew Crema Mexicana, is the perfect addition to any springtime party. In the cooler seasons, I like to use my Classic Red Enchilada Sauce (page 195) with this spinach and mushroom combo.

FOR THE FILLING
1 tablespoon vegetable oil
½ cup diced white or yellow onion
1 large garlic clove, minced
½ teaspoon ground cumin
1 cup white button mushrooms, sliced
3 cups spinach, stemmed and chopped
½ teaspoon salt
¼ teaspoon freshly ground black pepper

FOR THE ENCHILADAS
1 tablespoon vegetable oil
8 corn tortillas
3 cups Roasted Tomatillo Salsa (page 201)
¼ cup Cashew Crema Mexicana (page 230)
½ cup diced onion
½ cup chopped cilantro

1. **TO MAKE THE FILLING:** In a large skillet, heat the oil on medium-high heat. Add the onion, garlic, and cumin, and sauté until the onions are translucent.

2. Add the mushrooms and sauté, stirring occasionally, until they are lightly browned.

3. Add the spinach, salt, and pepper, and cook until almost all the liquid has evaporated. Remove from the heat.

1. **TO MAKE THE ENCHILADAS:** Preheat the oven to 350°F.

2. In a skillet, heat the oil and lightly pan-fry the tortillas until tender and pliable. Drain on a paper towel–lined plate. Repeat until all the tortillas have been panfried.

3. Spread ½ cup of Roasted Tomatillo Salsa in the bottom of a 9-by-13-inch baking dish and dip each tortilla into the sauce. Place the sauced tortillas on a plate and spoon about 1½ to 2 tablespoons of spinach and mushroom filling down the center of each tortilla. Roll up each tortilla and place seam side down in the baking dish. Repeat until all the tortillas are filled. Pour the remaining Roasted Tomatillo Salsa over the filled tortillas.

4. Bake the enchiladas for 15 minutes.

5. Top with Cashew Crema Mexicana, diced onion, and cilantro, and serve hot.

ORIGIN STORY: Enchiladas were originally called *chīllapītzalli*, which comes from the Nahuatl words *chīlli* (chile) and *tlapītzalli* (flute). Nahuatl is the language of the Aztecs.

COOKING TIP: For an extra punch of color and flavor, serve these enchiladas topped with quick pickled red onions instead of the diced white onion. To make the pickles, simply cover 1 peeled, slivered red onion in 1 cup water, ½ cup apple cider vinegar, and 1 tablespoon each sugar and salt. Let sit for at least 15 minutes.

SPICED POTATO ENCHILADAS

MAKES 8 ENCHILADAS • PREP TIME: 10 MINUTES • COOK TIME: 45 MINUTES

The word enchilada *comes from the Spanish word* enchilar, *which means "to season with chili." This recipe, featuring my classic red chile sauce, was a family favorite during the Lenten season. I have fond memories of jumping off the school bus on Friday afternoons and walking into Grandma's kitchen to the wonderful smell of these spiced potato–filled flutes. It always meant the weekend was off to a great start.*

FOR THE FILLING
1 tablespoon vegetable oil
½ cup diced white or yellow onion
1 large garlic clove, minced
½ teaspoon whole cumin seeds
1 large russet potato, peeled and
    diced small
¼ teaspoon chipotle powder
⅛ teaspoon cayenne powder
½ teaspoon dried Mexican oregano
½ teaspoon salt, plus more for
    seasoning
½ cup water

FOR THE ENCHILADAS
1 tablespoon vegetable oil
8 corn tortillas
3 cups Classic Red Enchilada Sauce
    (page 195), divided
1 cup vegan shredded white cheese
½ cup diced onion
½ cup chopped cilantro

1. **TO MAKE THE FILLING:** In a large skillet, heat the oil on medium-high heat. Add the onion, garlic, and cumin, and sauté until the onion is caramelized.

2. Add the potato, chipotle and cayenne powders, oregano, salt, and water, and mix well. Cover the skillet and reduce the heat to medium-low. Simmer until the potato is tender, about 15 minutes, stirring occasionally. Add a little more water if it seems to be sticking to the pan or drying out.

3. Remove from the heat and mash with a potato masher. Season again with salt and set aside.

1. **TO MAKE THE ENCHILADAS:** Preheat the oven to 350°F.

2. In a skillet, heat the oil and lightly pan-fry the tortillas until tender and pliable. Drain on a paper towel–lined plate. Repeat until all the tortillas have been panfried.

3. Spread ½ cup of Classic Red Enchilada Sauce in the bottom of a 9-by-13-inch baking dish and dip each tortilla into the sauce. Place the sauced tortillas on a plate and spoon about 2 tablespoons of the potato filling down the center of each tortilla. Roll up each tortilla and place seam side down in the baking dish. Repeat until all the tortillas are filled. Pour the remaining Classic Red Enchilada Sauce over the filled tortillas and top with cheese.

4. Bake the enchiladas for 15 to 20 minutes, or until the cheese is melted.

5. Top with diced onion and cilantro and serve hot.

SIMPLE SWAP: Sweet potatoes work wonderfully well for a sweeter version of this dish. Give them a try! Cooking time remains the same.

ENMOLADAS VERDES
WITH CHICKEN-STYLE SETAS

MAKES 8 EMMOLADAS • PREP TIME: 10 MINUTES • COOK TIME: 25 MINUTES

So we've covered enchiladas. What are these enmoladas all about? Enmoladas are similar to enchiladas, except they're topped with a mole sauce, while enchiladas are topped with a chile sauce. For this recipe, tender sautéed oyster mushrooms are matched up with a bright and fresh green mole sauce. This lighter take on classic chicken enmoladas is a weekend brunch favorite at Casa Garza.

FOR THE FILLING
1 tablespoon vegetable oil
½ cup diced small white or
   yellow onion
1 large garlic clove, minced
1 teaspoon cumin seeds, ground in
   a molcajete
¾ pound oyster mushrooms, chopped
½ teaspoon salt

FOR THE EMMOLADAS
1 tablespoon vegetable oil
8 corn tortillas
3 cups Green Mole (page 197),
   warmed, divided
¼ cup Cashew Crema Mexicana
   (page 230)
½ cup chopped cilantro

1. TO MAKE THE FILLING: In a large skillet, heat the oil on medium-high heat. Add the onion, garlic, and cumin, and sauté until the onions are translucent.

2. Add the mushrooms and salt. Sauté, stirring occasionally, until the mushrooms are cooked through and even in color.

3. Remove from the heat and set aside.

1. TO MAKE THE ENMOLADAS: In a skillet, heat the oil and lightly panfry the tortillas until tender and pliable. Drain on a paper towel–lined plate. Repeat until all the tortillas have been panfried.

2. Spread ½ cup of warm Green Mole sauce in the bottom of a 9-by-13-inch baking dish and dip each tortilla into the sauce. Place the sauced tortillas on a plate and spoon about 2 tablespoons of filling down the center of each tortilla. Roll up each tortilla and place seam side down in the baking dish. Repeat until all tortillas are filled.

3. Pour the remaining Green Mole sauce over filled tortillas and drizzle with Cashew Crema Mexicana. Top with cilantro and serve hot.

SIMPLE SWAP: Feel free to substitute your favorite plant-based chicken, shredded or small chopped, for the oyster mushrooms.

CHICKEN-STYLE SETAS MOLE

Learning to cook certain traditional dishes is almost like a rite of passage in many Mexican families. A friend of mine from the city of Monterrey jokingly comments on my Instagram posts with the phrase "ya te puedes casar" (meaning, "you can now get married") whenever I share pics of any those special dishes. Among those dishes are tamales, empanadas and, of course, mole. For this plant-based version of the Mexican classic, I simmer chicken-style oyster mushrooms in my easy Brown Mole.

2 teaspoons vegetable oil

2 pounds oyster mushrooms, roughly chopped

1 red onion, diced medium

1 red bell pepper, seeded and diced medium

1 serrano chile, seeded and minced

½ teaspoon salt

½ teaspoon freshly ground black pepper

2 cups Brown Mole (page 196)

Toasted sesame seeds

½ cup chopped red onion

1. Heat the oil in a medium saucepan on medium-high heat. Sauté the mushrooms for 5 to 7 minutes, or until well browned and they begin to release their juices. Add the onion, bell pepper, serrano chile, salt, and pepper and sauté for about 5 minutes more.

2. Pour in the Brown Mole sauce and bring to a boil. Reduce the heat to a simmer and cook, covered, for 20 minutes, stirring as needed so the mole does not burn.

3. To serve, spoon into bowls and top with sesame seeds and chopped red onion.

COOKING TIP: This *plato fuerte* (main dish) can be enjoyed on its own or as a hearty taco filling. It's a saucy dish, so serve it alongside Arroz Rojo (page 163) and corn or flour tortillas to help soak up all the delicious mole.

SEITAN ENCHILADAS SUIZAS

MAKES 8 ENCHILADAS • PREP TIME: 15 MINUTES • COOK TIME: 30 MINUTES

When we think of European influence on Mexican cuisine, the first country that might come to mind is Spain. However, Enchiladas Suizas came from Swiss immigrants, who brought cows to Mexico to set up dairies. Thankfully for you and for bovines, you don't need to be Swiss or enlist any cows to make this creamy classic. These Enchiladas Suizas are filled with cheesy seitan and topped with a decadent pink sauce that will have dinner guests begging for more.

FOR THE SWISS SAUCE
1 (15-ounce) can diced tomatoes, not drained
1 medium jalapeño chile, seeded
1 cup Cashew Crema Mexicana (page 230)

FOR THE FILLING
1½ tablespoons canola oil
½ small onion, diced
½ medium poblano chile, diced
1 teaspoon ground cumin
2 large garlic cloves, minced

1 cup chopped Mexican Seasoned Seitan (page 239)
¾ cup vegan shredded white cheese, divided
Salt
Freshly ground black pepper

FOR THE ENCHILADAS
1 tablespoon vegetable oil
8 corn tortillas
½ cup diced red onion

1. TO MAKE THE SWISS SAUCE: In a blender or food processor, combine the tomatoes and their juice, jalapeño, and Cashew Crema Mexicana.

2. Process until smooth and set aside.

1. TO MAKE THE FILLING: In a large skillet, heat the oil on medium heat. Sauté the onion until it is almost translucent. Add the poblano chile, cumin, and garlic, and sauté until the chile turns bright green.

2. Add the Mexican Seasoned Seitan and increase the heat to medium-high. Cook, stirring constantly, for about 5 minutes or until the seitan is nicely browned.

3. Add about ½ cup of the Swiss sauce and half the shredded cheese. Mix thoroughly until the cheese is mostly melted. Remove the skillet from the heat. Season with salt and pepper.

1. TO MAKE THE ENCHILADAS: Preheat the oven to 350°F.

2. In a skillet, heat the oil and lightly panfry the tortillas until tender and pliable. Drain on a paper towel–lined plate. Repeat until all the tortillas have been panfried.

3. Spread ½ cup of the Swiss sauce in the bottom of a 9-by-13-inch baking dish and dip each tortilla into the sauce. Place the sauced tortillas on a plate and spoon about 2 tablespoons of seitan filling down the center of each tortilla. Roll up each tortilla and place seam side down in the baking dish. Repeat until all the tortillas are filled. Pour the remaining sauce over the filled tortillas and top with the rest of the cheese.

4. Bake the enchiladas for 15 to 20 minutes, or until the cheese is melted.

5. Top with diced red onion and serve hot.

SIMPLE SWAP: I like to use seitan for these hearty enchiladas because it really holds the rich, creamy filling well. If you want a gluten-free version, simply replace the seitan with reconstituted TVP.

GRILLED CHIMICHURRI TOFU STEAKS
WITH PEPPERS AND ONIONS

**MAKES 4 STEAKS • PREP TIME: 10 MINUTES, PLUS 30 MINUTES TO MARINATE
COOK TIME: 10 MINUTES**

Like pesto, chimichurri sauce is one of those simple herb-based sauces that can make anything taste like a five-star meal. When I first went vegetarian, one of my go-to meals was grilled tofu chimichurri. It remains a favorite and is always one of the first items to disappear at my summer grilling parties. The trick is to let the tofu cutlets marinate in chimichurri for at least half an hour before grilling on a direct flame. The steaks are then nestled on a bed of grilled red pepper and onion and lathered with another coating of spicy chimichurri sauce. The end result is a smoky "steak" dinner that will have even your most carnivorous guests licking their plates clean.

1 cup Spicy Chimichurri (page 193)
1 (1-pound) package extra-firm tofu, sliced into 4 steaks
1 red bell pepper, cut in half, seeded
2 jalapeño chiles, halved lengthwise

1 red onion, sliced ½-inch thick
2 teaspoons vegetable oil
½ teaspoon salt
½ teaspoon freshly ground black pepper

1. Put the Spicy Chimichurri in a large bowl and add the tofu, bell pepper, jalapeños, onion, oil, salt, and pepper. Marinate in the refrigerator for at least 30 minutes to 1 hour. (Longer is always better.) Save the marinade to be served warmed on the side with the finished dish.

2. Shake off the extra marinade from the tofu (the oil in the sauce can cause the grill to flame up).

3. Grill the tofu, peppers, and onions on a direct flame over high heat, about 4 to 5 minutes on each side. Or cook in a hot cast-iron skillet.

4. To serve, slice the grilled tofu steaks on the bias, and serve on a bed of the pepper and onion. Serve with the warmed Spicy Chimichurri on the side or drizzled on top.

COOKING TIP: If you're cooking indoors, use a cast-iron skillet on medium-high heat to get a nice brown crust on the tofu and pepper and onion. Sear them all about 3 to 4 minutes on each side.

TOFU STEAK VERACRUZANA

MAKES 4 STEAKS • PREP TIME: 10 MINUTES, PLUS 30 MINUTES TO 1 HOUR MARINATING TIME • COOK TIME: 30 MINUTES

The cuisine of Veracruz is unlike any other in Mexico. It's a fusion of indigenous, Spanish, and Afro-Cuban flavors. Like all of Mexico, staple crops include corn, beans, squash, and chiles, but the dishes of Veracruz are uniquely characterized by the incorporation of a variety of tropical fruits and European ingredients like capers and olives. For this quick and easy dish a la Veracruzana, I combine seared tofu cutlets in a classic Veracruz-style tomato, white wine, capers, and olive salsa.

1 (1-pound) package extra-firm tofu, sliced into 4 steaks
2 garlic cloves, minced, divided
¼ cup Homemade Vegetable Stock (page 231)
1 teaspoon dried Mexican oregano
½ teaspoon salt, plus more for seasoning
½ teaspoon freshly ground black pepper, plus more for seasoning
Juice of 1 lime

2 teaspoons vegetable oil
1 red onion, julienned
1 jalapeño chile, seeded and julienned
1 red bell pepper, seeded and julienned
1 (3.5-ounce) jar capers, drained, rinsed, and roughly chopped
⅓ cup green olives, roughly chopped
3 Roma tomatoes, seeded and sliced very thin
¼ cup white wine
1 tablespoon vegan butter

1. Combine the tofu, 1 minced garlic clove, Homemade Vegetable Stock, oregano, salt, pepper, and lime juice in a large bowl. Marinate in the refrigerator for at least 30 minutes to 1 hour.

2. Heat a cast-iron skillet on medium-high heat and add the oil. Sear the tofu for about 5 to 7 minutes on each side, or until well browned. Remove from pan and set aside.

3. In the same pan, sauté the onion, jalapeño, and bell pepper for about 4 minutes. Add the capers, olives, and 1 minced garlic clove. Sauté 3 minutes.

4. Add the tomatoes and white wine. Reduce the heat to a simmer and add the tofu back into the pan. Cook down the sauce for about 5 minutes.

5. When sauce is reduced, stir in the butter, and season with salt and pepper.

6. Serve with the tofu sliced on the bias, covered with sauce and vegetables.

COOKING TIP: Grilling the tofu is another option for this dish. The sauce will still need to be made in a skillet, but it comes together quickly if you have the ingredients ready to go.

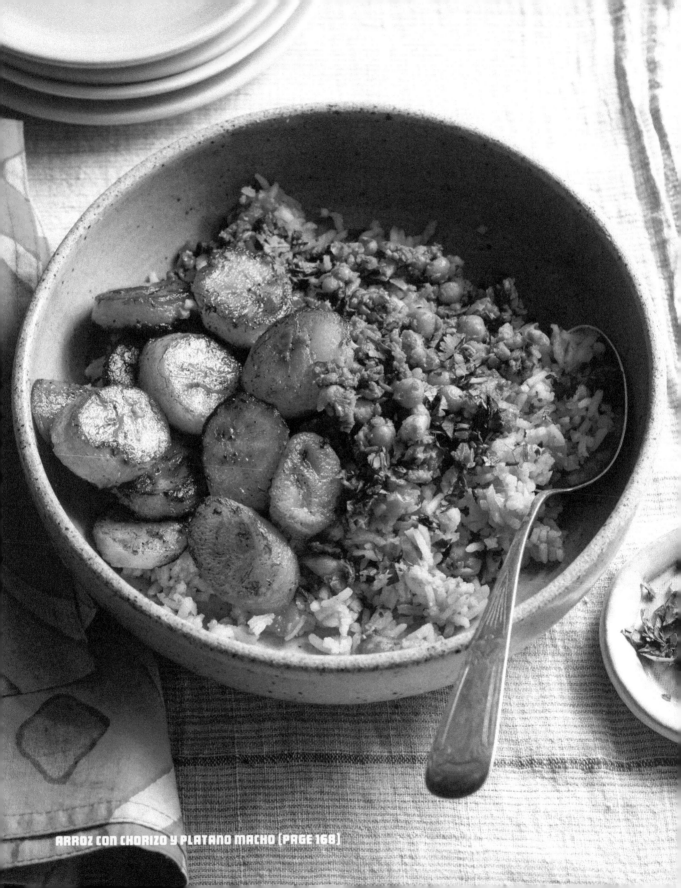

ARROZ CON CHORIZO Y PLATANO MACHO (PAGE 168)

Chapter 7

RICE, BEANS, AND SIDES

CILANTRO LIME RICE

MAKES ABOUT 4 CUPS • PREP TIME: 10 MINUTES • COOK TIME: 30 MINUTES

Cilantro lime rice is a popular sidekick to any Mexican dish and is also a satisfying solo delight. Do your taste buds a favor and be sure to use fresh cilantro and lime, if you can. Although you can use jasmine, basmati, long-grain, or short-grain rice in this simple recipe, I prefer long-grain white rice. Let the zest of flavor from fresh ingredients dance in your mouth as you reach for another bite.

FOR THE SAUCE
2 cups spinach
½ bunch cilantro
3 garlic cloves
Juice of 2 limes
1 teaspoon ground cumin
½ teaspoon salt
½ teaspoon freshly ground
    black pepper
¼ cup olive oil

FOR THE RICE
2 tablespoons vegetable oil
2 cups long-grain white rice
½ cup diced small white or
    yellow onion
2 garlic cloves, minced
½ teaspoon ground cumin
4 cups Homemade Vegetable
    Stock (page 231)
Salt
2 tablespoons chopped cilantro

1. TO MAKE THE SAUCE: Place all the ingredients except the oil into the bowl of a food processor and process until minced.

2. Slowly dribble in the oil and process until the mixture is smooth. Set aside.

1. TO MAKE THE RICE: In a large skillet, heat the oil over medium heat. Add the rice and sauté until it is slightly browned, about 5 minutes, stirring frequently to brown evenly. Add the onion, garlic, and cumin and sauté for another 1 to 2 minutes, stirring constantly.

2. Add the Homemade Vegetable Stock, season with salt, and bring to a boil. Cover and reduce the heat to medium-low. Simmer for about 15 to 20 minutes, or until all the liquid has been absorbed by the rice.

3. Remove from the heat.

4. Fold the sauce and fresh cilantro into the rice.

COOKING TIP: This dish is best served fresh. Maintain the beautiful bright green color by serving it right after you fold in the fresh cilantro and sauce.

ARROZ ROJO

MAKES ABOUT 4 CUPS • PREP TIME: 10 MINUTES • COOK TIME: 30 MINUTES

Arroz Rojo—meaning "red rice"—is a popular rice dish throughout northern Mexico and the Southwest. It's commonly referred to as Spanish rice in states along the Mexican border, though it's not recognized by that name in Mexico and the dish is largely unknown in Spain. Just like the noodles in Sopa de Fideo (page 57), the rice is lightly toasted before the stock is added to give it a nice nuttiness. This basic rice dish is the perfect accompaniment to any meal—from enchiladas to fajitas y más.

2 tablespoons vegetable oil
2 cups long-grain white rice
½ cup diced small white or
  yellow onion
2 garlic cloves, minced
½ teaspoon ground cumin

½ cup diced canned tomatoes
4 cups Homemade Vegetable
  Stock (page 231)
1 teaspoon fresh lime juice
Salt
¼ cup chopped cilantro

1. In a large skillet, heat the oil on medium heat, then sauté the rice until slightly browned, about 5 minutes, stirring constantly to brown evenly. Add the onion, garlic, and cumin and sauté for another 1 to 2 minutes, stirring constantly.

2. Add the tomatoes, Homemade Vegetable Stock, and lime juice, and season with salt. Bring to a boil, then simmer on medium-low heat, covered, for about 15 to 20 minutes, or until all liquid has been absorbed by the rice. Remove from the heat.

3. Top the rice with cilantro and use a fork to fluff the rice and combine the cilantro.

COOKING TIP: For a deeper colored rice, mix in a dollop of tomato paste with the vegetable stock.

ARROZ ENCHILADO

MAKES ABOUT 4 CUPS • PREP TIME: 10 MINUTES • COOK TIME: 30 MINUTES

Arroz Enchilado is another popular red rice dish enjoyed throughout northern Mexico. This spicier version of my classic Arroz Rojo (page 163) gets its red hue from guajillo, ancho, and árbol chile paste, which is lightly toasted with the rice before being simmered. Chipotle powder and dark chili powder are added to kick up the heat a bit. Use this base recipe for a spiced-up version of Arroz sin Pollo (page 166).

2 tablespoons vegetable oil
2 cups long-grain white rice
½ cup diced white or yellow onion
1 garlic clove, minced
½ teaspoon ground cumin
1 teaspoon dark chili powder
1 teaspoon chipotle powder

2 tablespoons Classic Chile Paste (page 194)
4 cups Homemade Vegetable Stock (page 231)
1 teaspoon fresh lime juice
Salt
¼ cup chopped cilantro

1. In a large skillet, heat the oil on medium heat, then sauté the rice until slightly browned, about 5 minutes, stirring constantly to brown evenly. Add the onion, garlic, and cumin and sauté for another 1 to 2 minutes, stirring constantly.

2. Add the chili powder, chipotle powder, and Classic Chile Paste and combine well. Add the Homemade Vegetable Stock and lime juice, and season with salt.

3. Bring to a boil, then simmer on medium-low heat, covered, for about 15 to 20 minutes or until all liquid has been absorbed by the rice. Remove from the heat.

4. Top the rice with cilantro and use a fork to fluff the rice and combine the cilantro.

HEAT INDEX: I love using chipotle powder in this recipe because of its wonderful smokiness and mild spice level. For an even spicier rice, add in a pinch of cayenne pepper. Just be careful not to overdo it—a little goes a long way!

MEXICAN WHITE RICE
WITH PEAS, CARROTS, AND CELERY

MAKES ABOUT 4 CUPS • PREP TIME: 10 MINUTES • COOK TIME: 30 MINUTES

A hearty side dish packed with goodness, this Mexican staple is as nutritious as it is delicious. Mexican white rice with peas, carrots, and celery is a versatile mainstay that's perfect to round out your traditional meal. There are many variations on this healthy side dish, so feel free to get creative—or stay true to this charming basic.

2 tablespoons vegetable oil
2 cups long-grain white rice
½ cup diced small white or
   yellow onion
2 garlic cloves, minced
¼ cup peeled and diced carrots
¼ cup diced celery

1 serrano chile, seeded and minced
4 cups Homemade Vegetable Stock
   (page 231)
¼ teaspoon salt
¼ teaspoon freshly ground
   black pepper
¼ cup frozen peas, thawed

1. In a large skillet, heat the oil on medium heat. Add the rice and sauté until slightly browned, about 5 minutes, stirring frequently to brown evenly. Add the onion, garlic, carrots, celery, and serrano chile, and sauté for another 4 minutes, stirring constantly.

2. Add the Homemade Vegetable Stock, salt, and pepper and bring to a boil. Cover and reduce the heat to medium-low. Simmer for about 15 to 20 minutes or until all liquid has been absorbed by the rice.

3. In the last 2 minutes of cooking, stir in the peas.

SIMPLE SWAP: For a Southwestern spin on this dish, replace the peas with frozen corn, the carrots with black beans, and the celery with butternut squash, diced small.

ARROZ SIN POLLO

MAKES ABOUT 4 CUPS • PREP TIME: 10 MINUTES • COOK TIME: 35 MINUTES

Dating back to Moorish Spain, Arroz con Pollo (rice with chicken) is a classic rice dish popular in all Latin American cuisine. Of course, every region has its own rendition, based on available ingredients. For this meat-free version of one of my childhood faves, I sauté shredded oyster mushrooms in place of chicken, then toss them in as a meaty ingredient with my classic Arroz Rojo (page 163). This method of preparation will have even your most meat-loving guests asking for seconds.

½ pound oyster mushrooms
3 tablespoons vegetable oil, divided
½ teaspoon salt, plus more
  for seasoning
Freshly ground black pepper
2 cups long-grain white rice
½ cup diced small white or
  yellow onion
2 garlic cloves, minced

1 jalapeño chile, seeded and minced
½ teaspoon ground cumin
1 (15-ounce) can diced tomatoes,
  drained
4 cups Homemade Vegetable
  Stock (page 231)
1 teaspoon fresh lime juice
¼ bunch cilantro, chopped

1. Shred the oyster mushrooms by hand.

2. In a large skillet, heat 1 tablespoon of oil on medium-high heat, then sauté the mushrooms for about 7 minutes, or until browned. Season with salt and pepper, transfer to a bowl, and set aside.

3. In the same skillet, heat the remaining 2 tablespoons of oil on medium heat, then sauté the rice until slightly browned, about 5 minutes, stirring constantly to brown evenly. Add the onion, garlic, jalapeño, and cumin, and sauté for another 1 to 2 minutes, stirring constantly.

4. Add the tomatoes, Homemade Vegetable Stock, mushrooms, lime juice, and ½ teaspoon of salt. Bring to a boil, then simmer on medium-low heat, covered, for about 15 to 20 minutes or until all liquid has been absorbed by the rice.

5. Remove from the heat. Top the rice with cilantro and use a fork to fluff the rice and combine the cilantro.

SIMPLE SWAP: Prepared in this fashion, oyster mushrooms have the soft texture of dark cuts of chicken. If you prefer a meatier texture, try using chicken-style seitan or your favorite brand of plant-based chicken strips.

ARROZ con FRIJOLES NEGROS

MAKES ABOUT 4 CUPS • PREP TIME: 10 MINUTES • COOK TIME: 35 MINUTES

A power duo loved by cultures around the world, rice and beans are one of the most perfect food combinations. Together, they provide enough energy to serve as a whole meal. For this protein-rich bowl, we combine rice with the Mexican-native black bean and an array of Mexican seasonings. Any hearty bean works wonderfully in this dish. Try replacing the black beans with native Mexican varieties, like pintos or Peruanos.

2 tablespoons vegetable oil
2 cups long-grain white rice
½ cup diced white or yellow onion
2 garlic cloves, minced
½ teaspoon ground cumin
1 chipotle chile, canned in adobo, minced
4 cups Homemade Vegetable Stock (page 231)

2 teaspoons fresh lime juice
1½ teaspoons dried Mexican oregano
½ teaspoon salt
½ teaspoon freshly ground black pepper
1 (15-ounce) can black beans, drained and rinsed
¼ bunch cilantro, chopped

1. In a large skillet, heat the oil on medium heat, then sauté the rice until slightly browned, about 5 minutes, stirring constantly to brown evenly. Add the onion, garlic, cumin, and chipotle chile, and sauté for another 1 to 2 minutes, stirring constantly.

2. Add the Homemade Vegetable Stock, lime juice, oregano, salt, and pepper. Bring to a boil, then simmer on medium-low heat, covered, for about 15 to 20 minutes or until all liquid has been absorbed by the rice. Stir in the black beans in the last 2 to 4 minutes of cooking. Remove from the heat.

3. Top the rice with cilantro and use a fork to fluff the rice and combine the cilantro.

ORIGIN STORY: Rice was introduced into Mexico by Spanish settlers in the 1520s. Since then, it has been a staple in Mexican cuisine.

ARROZ con CHORIZO Y PLATANO MACHO

MAKES ABOUT 4 CUPS • PREP TIME: 10 MINUTES • COOK TIME: 15 MINUTES

At Casa Garza growing up, we never let anything go to waste, including leftover rice. My father used to sauté it with other ingredients to make bulky rice bowls. (Dad likes to think he invented the burrito bowl, but he might think the same of most of Taco Bell's menu.) One of my favorite rice bowls Dad made consisted of leftover Arroz Rojo (page 163), spicy chorizo, and ripe, sweet plantains. For this vegan version, I'm using my chickpea-based Garbanzorizo, which packs a protein punch and just the right amount of heat. It's a flavor combination that always takes me way back.

2 tablespoons vegetable oil
1 ripe plantain, peeled and sliced
¼ teaspoon salt
¼ teaspoon freshly ground
   black pepper

1 cup Garbanzorizo (page 242)
2 cups Arroz Rojo (page 163)
1 teaspoon fresh lime juice

1. In a large skillet, heat the oil on medium-high heat. Sauté the plantain for about 7 minutes, or until browned and soft. Sprinkle with the salt and pepper.

2. Stir in the Garbonzorizo and sauté for 4 more minutes.

3. Fold in the Arroz Rojo and heat through.

4. Stir in the lime juice and serve.

SECRET INGREDIENT: Plantains are ripe when skin is dark yellow with lots of black patchy areas. To fast-ripen plantains, roast them skin-on at 300°F for 45 minutes. Let cool completely in the refrigerator before using.

ARROZ A LA TUMBADA

MAKES ABOUT 4 CUPS • PREP TIME: 15 MINUTES • COOK TIME: 30 MINUTES

When the Spaniards first brought rice to Mexico in the 1520s through the port of Veracruz—a tropical region with a warm, moist climate—they knew it would the ideal location for the cultivation of the grain that is now a staple in Mexican cuisine. Arroz a la Tumbada, a rice and seafood dish slightly soupier than Spanish seafood paella, quickly became one of Veracruz's signature dishes. For this plant-based version of the popular soupy rice, I use sliced hearts of palm, quartered artichoke hearts, and dulse flakes to give this dish a fresh sea flavor without the fish.

2 tablespoons vegetable oil
2 cups long-grain white rice
½ white onion, julienned
2 garlic cloves, minced
½ teaspoon ground cumin
2 guajillo chiles, rehydrated in hot water for 15 minutes, seeded, stemmed, and chopped
1 (14-ounce) can whole hearts of palm, drained, sliced ½ inch thick on the bias

5 cups Homemade Vegetable Stock (page 231)
1 tablespoon dulse flakes
2 teaspoons fresh lime juice
½ teaspoon salt
½ teaspoon freshly ground black pepper
1 (14-ounce) can whole artichoke hearts, drained, quartered
Lime wedges, for garnish

1. In a large skillet, heat the oil on medium heat, then sauté the rice until slightly browned, about 5 minutes, stirring constantly to brown evenly. Add the onion, garlic, cumin, guajillo chiles, and hearts of palm and sauté for another 2 to 4 minutes, stirring constantly.

2. Add the Homemade Vegetable Stock, dulse flakes, lime juice, salt, and pepper. Evenly distribute the artichoke hearts over the rice. Bring to a boil, then simmer on medium-low heat, covered, for about 15 to 20 minutes. Remove from the heat.

3. Serve hot with a lime wedge.

COOKING TIP: This rice dish should be a little soupy. For a more traditional rice style, simply cut back the amount of vegetable stock to 4 cups and simmer until all the liquid has been absorbed by the rice.

ARROZ con NOPALES

MAKES ABOUT 4 CUPS • PREP TIME: 10 MINUTES • COOK TIME: 15 MINUTES

I have fond memories of taking weekday bus trips with my grandma to visit my great-grandmother during summer breaks. My great-grandma lived in a small house on the edge of the city (her house was literally steps from the Mexican border), and I loved playing outside in her backyard, which was lined with rose bushes and nopal cactuses. Lunchtime at great-grandma's always included nopales in some form or fashion, and one of my favorites was Arroz con Nopales. For this nostalgic rice recipe, I've prepared it just like great-grandma did. She always preboiled and drained the nopales to get rid of some of the cactus's natural gooeyness, then sautéed them with a little onion, garlic, and leftover Arroz Rojo. Simple and delicious!

4 cups water
¾ teaspoon salt, divided
2 nopal cactus pads, dethorned, peeled, and diced medium
2 tablespoons vegetable oil
½ white onion, julienned

2 garlic cloves, minced
¼ teaspoon freshly ground black pepper
2 cups Arroz Rojo (page 163)
1 teaspoon fresh lime juice

1. In a large pot, bring the water and ½ teaspoon of salt to a boil. Add the nopales and boil for about 5 to 7 minutes. Drain and rinse in a colander.

2. In a large skillet, heat the oil on medium-high heat and sauté the nopales and onion about 7 minutes or until almost all the *babas* (gooey liquid) from the cactus is gone. Add the garlic, pepper, and remaining ½ teaspoon salt, and sauté for 2 minutes more.

3. Fold in the Arroz Rojo and heat through. Stir in the lime juice and serve.

SECRET INGREDIENT: Nopales are super low in fat, high in fiber, and high in vitamin C, with amazing anti-inflammatory properties. Add this meaty cactus to bulk up any dish.

REFRIED BLACK BEANS

SERVES 8 • PREP TIME: 5 MINUTES • COOK TIME: 25 MINUTES

Also known as turtle beans, Mexican beans, and Tampico beans, black beans have been a long time staple in Mexican cuisine—and for good reason. They're packed with protein, fiber, and antioxidants, and they're absolutely delicious any way you cook them. In this refried black bean recipe, onion and garlic are caramelized before the beans are added, to bring a deep complexity to the dish. Use this recipe for filling tlacoyos or sopes, or enjoy on their own as a snack (topped with a little avocado, naturally).

1 tablespoon vegetable oil
½ cup diced white onion
3 garlic cloves, minced
1 to 2 serrano chiles, minced
1 tablespoon ground cumin
1 tablespoon chili powder

2 (15-ounce) cans black beans,
    1 drained and rinsed, 1 not drained
½ teaspoon salt
½ teaspoon freshly ground
    black pepper
Juice of 1 lime

1. In a medium saucepan, heat the oil on medium-high heat, then sauté the onion for 7 to 10 minutes. As the onion starts to brown, add the garlic, serrano chiles, cumin, and chili powder. Continue to sauté until the garlic and the onion gets nicely caramelized, about 12 minutes. They should be browned but not burned.

2. Add both cans of beans (with the liquid from one) and bring to a boil. Reduce the heat and simmer for 10 minutes.

3. Using an immersion blender (or in a standing blender), purée the beans for about 3 minutes. You want a nice consistency; some whole beans are fine, and the dish should not be smooth.

4. Mix in the salt, pepper, and lime juice.

5. Cook the beans to thicken, stirring as needed, for about 5 minutes.

HEAT INDEX: For slightly milder version of this dish, take the seeds out of the serranos before you add them. For an even milder version, omit them entirely.

BLACK BEAN ALBONDIGAS in CHIPOTLE RANCHERO SAUCE

MAKES 8 TO 10 BALLS • PREP TIME: 10 MINUTES • COOK TIME: 40 MINUTES

While beans are the nutritional powerhouse base of this recipe, the real star here is the tasty chipotles . . . but did you know they have a secret? Chipotle chiles are really just large jalapeños, dried and then smoked. This process creates a unique sweet-and-smoky flavor that shines in this versatile recipe. Toss these bean balls onto a small plate for an evening of tapas or—for a fun and spicy party appetizer—place a toothpick in each and watch your guests make them disappear!

1 (15-ounce) can black beans, drained and rinsed

1 cup rolled oats

½ cup Homemade Vegetable Stock (page 231) or water

4 tablespoons vital wheat gluten

2 tablespoons ground flaxseed, mixed with 6 tablespoons warm water

2 tablespoons nutritional yeast

1 tablespoon chopped cilantro

1 teaspoon ground cumin

1 teaspoon chili powder

1 teaspoon granulated garlic

½ teaspoon salt

½ teaspoon freshly ground black pepper

¼ teaspoon dried Mexican oregano

4 tablespoons vegetable oil

2 chipotle chiles, canned in adobo sauce, minced

3 cups Salsa Ranchera (page 199)

½ cup Almond Queso Cotija (page 73)

½ cup chopped cilantro, for garnish

1. Place the beans, oats, Homemade Vegetable Stock, wheat gluten, flaxseed and water, nutritional yeast, cilantro, cumin, chili powder, garlic, salt, pepper, and oregano in the blender.

2. Process for about 30 seconds, then scrape the sides down and process for about 30 seconds more. The mixture should resemble a thick and moist dough. If it is too wet, add 1 teaspoon of vital wheat gluten to the mix and pulse again.

3. Scrape the mixture into a bowl and set aside.

4. In a medium saucepan, heat the oil on medium-high heat. Scoop out meatballs with a small ice cream scoop, or use about 3 tablespoons at a time; shape each portion by hand into bean balls.

5. Fry the bean balls in the saucepan for about 5 minutes on each side, giving them time to get a nice brown sear to them.

6. Add the chipotles to the Salsa Ranchera and mix well. Pour the salsa in the pan with the albondigas. Bring to a boil. Reduce the heat to a simmer. Cover and cook for about 15 minutes.

7. To serve, scoop 3 bean balls and some sauce into a bowl, and garnish with Almond Queso Cotija and cilantro.

COOKING TIP: These albondigas can be baked too. Just use a mini muffin pan, lightly sprayed with oil. Scoop some bean mixture into the pan's cups. Bake at 350°F for 30 to 40 minutes, or until well browned. Then simmer in the sauce for about 10 minutes. These also make great bean ball subs; just toss 3 to 4 albondigas onto a freshly toasted bolillo and top with a mild vegan shredded cheese.

SPICY REFRIED PINTO BEANS

SERVES 8 • PREP TIME: 5 MINUTES • COOK TIME: 25 MINUTES

A traditional dish in both northern Mexican and Tex-Mex cuisine, refried pinto beans are made by cooking pintos, mashing them, then cooking them some more. This spicy rendition of the northern Mexican classic is a Garza family favorite. Use this recipe to stuff gorditas, top tostadas, or serve alongside your favorite Mexican rice dish. Remove the seeds from serranos if you want to reduce the heat a bit.

1 tablespoon vegetable oil
½ cup diced small white onion
3 garlic cloves, minced
1 to 2 serrano chiles, seeded and minced
1 tablespoon ground cumin
½ teaspoon dried Mexican oregano
1 tablespoon chili powder

2 (15-ounce) cans pinto beans, 1 drained and rinsed, 1 not drained
½ teaspoon salt
½ teaspoon freshly ground black pepper
Juice of 1 lime
3 tablespoons chopped cilantro

1. In a medium saucepan, heat the oil on medium-high heat, then sauté the onion for 5 to 7 minutes. As the onion start to get color, add the garlic, serrano chiles, cumin, oregano, and chili powder. Continue to sauté for 5 minutes more. The onion should be soft and the garlic browned.

2. Add both cans of beans (with the liquid from one) and bring to a boil. Reduce the heat and simmer for 10 minutes.

3. You want a nice consistency; some whole beans are fine, and the dish should not be smooth.

4. Spinkle with the salt, pepper, and lime juice.

5. Cook the beans to thicken, stirring as needed, for about 5 minutes.

6. Fold in the cilantro.

ORIGIN STORY: Friends often ask me why they're called "refried beans," since the beans aren't fried in the first place. The name of the dish comes from a literal translation of the Spanish "frijoles refritos." In Spanish, the prefix *re-* is used for emphasis, so "frijoles refritos" actually means "well-fried beans" (meaning cooked well), as opposed to "beans that are fried again."

BORRACHO BEANS WITH GREEN CHILES

SERVES 6 • PREP TIME: 15 MINUTES, PLUS OVERNIGHT SOAKING TIME • COOK TIME: 2 HOURS

Borracho beans are a style of Mexican charro beans (cowboy beans)—pinto beans stewed with onion, garlic, bacon, and, of course, beer. Borracho means "drunk." It's the perfect side dish for Refried Bean and Seitan Beef-Style Tostadas (page 97) and Arroz Rojo (page 163) or enjoyed all on its own.

1 pound dry pinto beans
1 tablespoon vegetable oil
1 medium white onion, diced small
1 (4-ounce) can diced green chiles
 or 2 fresh green chiles of your
 choice, diced
1 serrano chile, seeded and minced
¾ cup tempeh bacon or smoked tofu,
 diced small
4 garlic cloves, minced
4 Roma tomatoes, diced medium
1 tablespoon ground cumin

1 tablespoon dark chili powder
1 teaspoon salt
1 teaspoon freshly ground black pepper
1 teaspoon dried Mexican oregano
4 cups Homemade Vegetable Stock
 (page 231)
1½ cups Mexican dark beer
1 sprig fresh epazote, chopped
3 tablespoons chopped cilantro,
 plus ½ bunch chopped, for garnish
2 limes, quartered

1. In a large bowl, soak the beans overnight, covered by at least by 2 inches of water.

2. In a large stock pot, heat the oil on medium-high heat. Sauté the onion, green chiles, serrano chile, and tempeh bacon or smoked tofu for about 5 minutes. Add the garlic, tomatoes, cumin, chili powder, salt, pepper, and oregano. Sauté for 5 minutes. The onions should be soft and the tempeh should be browned.

3. Drain the beans and add to the pot, along with the Homemade Vegetable Stock, beer, and epazote. Bring to a boil, then reduce the heat to a simmer, cover, and cook for 1½ to 2 hours, stirring as needed. If the beans need a bit more liquid, add water or more stock, a cup or

so at a time. Adjust the seasoning as well. The beans should be cooked through and creamy when done.

4. In the last 5 minutes of cooking, add the cilantro. Serve garnished with more cilantro and lime wedges.

COOKING TIP: You can make this dish in a slow cooker. Follow steps 1 and 2, then transfer everything to the slow cooker and follow your cooker's directions for cooking the beans. If you are really pressed for time, you can make these using canned beans. Following steps 1 and 2, then add three (15-ounce) cans of pinto beans with their juice and omit the stock (but not the beer!). Cook uncovered for 10 to 15 minutes.

PERUANO BEANS WITH POBLANOS AND TOMATILLOS

SERVES 6 • PREP TIME: 15 MINUTES, PLUS OVERNIGHT SOAKING TIME • COOK TIME: 45 MINUTES

Despite their name, Peruano (Peruvian) beans are native to Mexico. These small, yellow oval beans have a wonderfully creamy texture when cooked. Also known as canary or Mayacoba beans, Peruanos are milder than black beans and are great at taking on any flavors you can throw at them while still maintaining their shape. In this recipe, Peruanos soak up the fresh flavors of poblano chiles and bright tomatillos. Enjoy these with your favorite tacos and tortas.

1 pound dry Peruano beans

1 tablespoon vegetable oil

1 medium white onion, diced small

2 fresh poblano chiles, seeded and diced small, or any other medium-heat green chiles

1 jalapeño chile, seeded and minced

3 celery stalks, diced small

1 medium carrot, peeled, diced small

4 garlic cloves, minced

6 fresh tomatillos, diced medium

1 tablespoon ground cumin

½ teaspoon whole cumin seeds

1 teaspoon ground coriander

1 teaspoon salt

1 teaspoon freshly ground black pepper

1 teaspoon dried Mexican oregano

4 cups Homemade Vegetable Stock (page 231)

1 sprig fresh epazote, chopped

Juice of 2 limes, plus 2 limes cut in quarters, for garnish

3 tablespoons minced cilantro, plus ½ bunch chopped, for garnish

1. In a large bowl, soak the beans overnight, covered at least by 2 inches of water.

2. In a large stock pot, heat the oil on medium-high heat, then sauté the onion, poblano and jalapeño chiles, celery, and carrot for about 5 minutes. Add the garlic, tomatillos, ground and whole cumin, coriander, salt, pepper, and oregano. Sauté for 5 minutes. The vegetables should be soft and the onion translucent.

3. Drain the beans and add to the pot, along with the Homemade Vegetable Stock and epazote. Bring to a boil, then reduce the heat to a simmer. Cover and cook for 30 to 45 minutes, stirring as needed. If the beans need a bit more liquid, add water or more Homemade Vegetable Stock, a cup or so at a time. Adjust the seasoning as well. The beans should be cooked through and creamy when done. In the last 5 minutes of cooking, add the lime juice and minced cilantro.

4. Serve with more cilantro and lime wedges.

COOKING TIP: Never hard-boil your beans; cooking them at a nice simmer will keep them whole and the creaminess will really come through. You can adapt this recipe for a slow cooker by using canned beans and following the instructions for Borracho Beans with Green Chiles (page 175).

MEXICAN-STYLE BEANS and GREENS

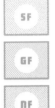

SF

GF

NF

Q&E

SERVES 4 • PREP TIME: 10 MINUTES • COOK TIME: 15 MINUTES

One of the many things I picture when I hear the words "comfort food" is a heaping bowl of hearty beans and greens. It's also one of the most affordable, healthy, and easy meals you can make—which is why you can find different versions of this one-dish meal all around the world. My Mexican-style recipe features pinto beans and Swiss chard—called acel- gas in Mexico—and it's spiced to perfection with serrano chile and dark chili powder. Curl up on the couch with this dish and your favorite guilty- pleasure TV show, and you have yourself the comfiest of comfort dinners.

1 tablespoon vegetable oil
½ white onion, diced small
1 serrano chile, seeded and minced
2 garlic cloves, minced
2 Roma tomatoes, diced medium
1 bunch Swiss chard, washed and
    roughly chopped

1 (15-ounce) can pinto beans,
    not drained
1 teaspoon ground cumin
1 teaspoon dark chili powder
½ teaspoon salt
½ teaspoon freshly ground
    black pepper

1. In a large skillet, heat the oil on medium-high heat, then sauté the onion and serrano chile for 5 minutes. Add the garlic, tomatoes, and chard, and sauté for 5 minutes more.

2. Stir in the beans with their liquid. Add the cumin and chili powder, and cook for 5 minutes, or until the beans are hot.

3. Mix with the salt and pepper and serve.

SIMPLE SWAP: Any combination of beans and hearty greens works great with this recipe. I love using chard because I have a ton of it growing in my garden, but kale is another wonderful option.

ROASTED BROCCOLI AND CAULIFLOWER

SERVES 4 TO 6 • PREP TIME: 10 MINUTES, PLUS 15 MINUTES SOAKING TIME •
COOK TIME: 20 MINUTES

When I was younger, my brother used to call broccoli and cauliflower "little trees," and it only makes sense to include in this book what is still one of our favorite dishes. This is perfect as a side for any dish, or as a small plate at a tapas-style meal. The roasting brings a welcome depth to the veggies, which are beautifully matched by the zip of the chile seasoning. They might look like little trees, but this dish packs big flavor.

2 heads broccoli, cut on sharp angles into florets with 1 to 3 inches of stem

1 head cauliflower, cut on sharp angles into florets

2 dried guajillo chiles, rehydrated in hot water for 15 minutes, seeded, stemmed, and chopped

3 garlic cloves, minced

2 tablespoons vegetable oil

2 teaspoons whole cumin seeds

Juice of 1 lime

½ teaspoon salt

½ teaspoon freshly ground black pepper

2 tablespoons chopped cilantro

1. Preheat the oven to 425°F.

2. In a large bowl, toss all the ingredients except the cilantro, and mix well with your hands. Spread out the vegetables on a large roasting pan.

3. Roast the veggies for 15 to 20 minutes, stirring halfway through the cooking time. The veggies should have nice brown color to the edges.

4. Remove from the oven and garnish with the chopped cilantro.

HEAT INDEX: To kick up the heat, use 2 to 4 chiles de árbol instead of the guajillo chiles. If you're in a time crunch, simply use crushed red chili flakes.

GRILLED MIXED VEGETABLES
WITH CHIMICHURRI

MAKES ABOUT 12 SKEWERS • PREP TIME: 20 MINUTES, PLUS 30 MINUTES MARINATING TIME • COOK TIME: 15 MINUTES

I'm a firm believer that the best meals are made from ingredients that travel the shortest distance between the ground and our plates. That's why I think of this dish as a gift from Mother Nature. Plants soak in the sun's rays, which provide the energy needed for herbs and vegetables to gather various nutrients from our planet's air, land, and water. Then we combine an array of flavors provided by each unique plant onto a skewer and heat them over an indispensable partner in our journey—an open flame. Savor each bite.

4 cups water
Ice
12 broccoli florets
12 cauliflower florets
2 medium zucchini, sliced ½ inch thick
2 medium yellow squash, sliced ½ inch thick
2 large red onions, cut into least 24 large pieces

2 large red bell peppers, cut into at least 12 pieces
12 button mushrooms
2 cups Spicy Chimichurri (page 193)
12 bamboo or wooden skewers, or reusable metal ones

1. In a medium saucepan, boil 4 cups of water to blanch the vegetables.

2. Meanwhile, fill a large bowl about halfway with ice and cold water to shock your blanched broccoli and cauliflower. This blanching process is fast, so have it set up ahead.

3. Add the broccoli to boiling water for about 2 minutes, until the florets become a vivid bright green. Quickly remove the florets from the pot with tongs or a small

hand strainer and immediately plunge them into the large bowl of ice water. Once chilled (about 2 minutes), remove them from the ice bath.

4. If needed, add more ice to your bowl for the next batch of veggies.

5. Repeat with the cauliflower. It should go from raw to blanched in about 2 to 3 minutes (remember the florets needs to hold their shape so they will skewer well).

6. Place the raw zucchini, squash, onions, bell peppers, mushrooms, and the blanched cauliflower and broccoli in a large bowl. Drench with Spicy Chimichurri and toss well. Cover and marinate in the refrigerator for at least 30 minutes.

7. Thread all the veggies on skewers, alternating them. I would suggest a pepper or onion on the bottom and a broccoli floret on top. This is a nice way to hold it all together.

8. Grill the skewers on a preheated grill over high direct heat for about 3 to 4 minutes on each side. You want all the veggies to get some char on them. Or broil on the middle-top rack of a broiler, on high setting, for 4 to 5 minutes, turning halfway through the cooking time.

9. To serve, stack on a large platter and pour the remaining marinade all over them.

COOKING TIP: When using wooden or bamboo skewers, soak them in water for about 10 minutes before use. This will prevent them from burning while you are grilling.

NOPALES GUISADOS

SERVES 6 • PREP TIME: 10 MINUTES • COOK TIME: 20 MINUTES

If you like Mediterranean-style stewed okra and tomatoes, you're going to love this Mexican nopales guisados recipe. Like okra, nopal cactus releases a silky, somewhat gooey liquid called babas *(which translates as "drool"); the acid of the tomatoes will balance it out. When stewed with rich tomatoes and savory vegetable stock, the nopales reach a wonderful flavor balance. And the aromas will literally have you drooling! Enjoy this guisado as a savory side dish or as a hearty topper for rice dishes.*

1 tablespoon canola oil

1 medium red onion, julienned

3 large nopal cactus pads, dethorned, peeled, and cut into 1-inch squares

1 garlic clove, minced

1 large jalapeño chile, seeded and diced

½ cup canned diced tomatoes, not drained

1 cup Homemade Vegetable Stock (page 231)

2 tablespoons chopped cilantro

½ teaspoon fresh lime juice

1 teaspoon ground cumin

½ teaspoon salt

¼ teaspoon freshly ground black pepper

1. In a large skillet, heat the oil on medium-high heat, then sauté the onion and nopales until the nopales are lightly browned and the onion is almost translucent. The mixture should be a little slimy.

2. Add the garlic and jalapeño and sauté until the jalapeño is bright green.

3. Add the tomatoes and some juice, Homemade Vegetable Stock, cilantro, lime juice, cumin, salt, and pepper.

4. Bring to a boil, then simmer, uncovered, for about 7 to 10 minutes, or until most of the liquid has evaporated.

5. Serve hot.

SECRET INGREDIENT: If cooking nopal cactus weirds you out because of its natural babas, here's an easy way get rid of most of it before starting this delicious guisado. Boil the nopales in a large pot for about 5 minutes, then drain and rinse in a colander. If you're using this method, add the nopales in step 2 of this recipe.

COOKING TIP: This recipe is Quick & Easy if you have vegetable stock on hand.

CREAMED CALABACITAS

SERVES 6 • PREP TIME: 10 MINUTES • COOK TIME: 15 MINUTES

The literal translation for calabacitas *is "squash." And it specifically refers to a small, pale green-skinned Mexican squash with yellow and white speckles. But the word* calabacitas *is also the name of this common side dish, which combines a medley of colors and flavors with the calabacita squash. For this recipe, red bell peppers, poblano chiles, corn, Cashew Crema Mexicana, and vegan cream cheese are tossed together to create a robust side dish.*

1 tablespoon vegetable oil
1 white onion, diced medium
1 red bell pepper, diced medium
2 garlic cloves, minced
1 cup frozen or fresh corn kernels
  (from about 2 ears of corn)
2 yellow squash, diced medium
2 calabacitas, diced medium
1 teaspoon ground cumin
1 poblano chile, charred or roasted,
  skinned, seeded and diced small

¼ cup Homemade Vegetable
  Stock (page 231)
½ teaspoon salt
½ teaspoon freshly ground
  black pepper
½ cup Cashew Crema Mexicana
  (page 230)
1 tablespoon vegan cream cheese
2 tablespoons chopped cilantro

1. In large, deep skillet, heat the oil on medium-high heat. Sauté the onion, bell pepper, and garlic for 3 minutes. Add the corn, squash, calabacitas, cumin, and poblano, and sauté for 3 minutes more.

2. Add the Homemade Vegetable Stock and the salt and pepper. Cover and reduce the heat. Simmer for about 10 minutes—less if you prefer firmer veggies.

3. Stir in the Cashew Crema Mexicana, cream cheese, and cilantro, and cook until the cream cheese is melted, stirring as needed.

4. Serve hot.

SIMPLE SWAP: This recipe is good with any summer squash. Try pattypan, sunburst, or zucchini. You can also add fresh tomatoes and omit the Cashew Crema Mexicana for a lower-fat option.

RAJAS con CREMA

A popular side dish at taquizas (taco parties) in central and southern Mexico, Rajas con Crema really bring the party to life. Rajas *means "slices" in Spanish. This dish features sliced poblano chiles sautéed with julienned onions, Cashew Crema Mexicana, a dab of vegan cream cheese, then a sprinkling of shredded vegan white cheese. It's the perfect accompaniment to any taco, torta, or Burritos Enmolados (page 130).*

1 tablespoon vegetable oil
1 white onion, julienned
2 garlic cloves, minced
6 poblano chiles, charred or roasted, peeled, seeded, and julienned
¼ cup Homemade Vegetable Stock (page 231)
½ teaspoon salt

½ teaspoon freshly ground black pepper
½ cup Cashew Crema Mexicana (page 230)
1 tablespoon vegan cream cheese
½ cup vegan shredded white cheese
2 tablespoons chopped cilantro

1. In large, deep skillet, heat the oil on medium-high heat. Sauté the onion and garlic for 4 minutes. Add the poblano chiles, Homemade Vegetable Stock, salt, and pepper.

2. Bring to a boil, then cover, reduce the heat, and simmer for about 5 minutes—or less if you prefer firmer veggies.

3. Stir in the Cashew Crema Mexicana and the cream cheese and cook until the cream cheese is blended in, stirring as needed.

4. To serve, garnish with shredded cheese and cilantro.

COOKING TIP: This recipe can be made in the oven. Sauté the onion and garlic, then place everything but the shredded cheese and cilantro in a medium casserole dish and bake at 350°F for 15 to 20 minutes (or until the mixture is bubbling and slightly brown on top). Remove from the oven and sprinkle on the cheese, then place back in the oven to brown the cheese, about 5 minutes. Garnish with cilantro and serve.

COOKING TIP: If you have vegetable stock ready, this recipe comes together in just 20 minutes.

WINTER HOLIDAY ROASTED HARD SQUASH

SERVES 4 • PREP TIME: 20 MINUTES • COOK TIME: 1 HOUR

Looking for a no-frills side dish for your Mexican winter holiday dinner? This roasted squash dish is just the thing. And bonus—squash is loaded with fiber and packed with nutrients such as vitamin A, beta-carotene, calcium, and potassium. Especially tempting in the colder months, this warm winter side is as festive as it is filling. With hints of cinnamon, thyme, and coriander, my Winter Holiday Roasted Hard Squash is hearty enough to serve as a main dish or can perfectly accompany your winter spread.

Nonstick cooking spray
1 butternut squash, peeled, seeded, and diced medium
1 red onion, diced medium
2 tablespoons brown sugar
1 tablespoon fresh lime juice

¼ teaspoon ground cinnamon
¼ teaspoon dried thyme
⅛ teaspoon ground coriander
¼ teaspoon salt
2 tablespoons vegan butter, melted
½ cup Aztec Spiced Pepitas (page 69)

1. Preheat the oven to 350°F. Lightly spray a large roasting pan with nonstick cooking spray.

2. In a large bowl, mix everything except the Aztec Spiced Pepitas. Mix well with your hands until everything is coated nicely with the spices and melted butter.

3. Roast, uncovered, 50 minutes to 1 hour. The squash is done when it is soft and slightly brown, and the onions will be caramelized.

4. Garnish with Aztec Spiced Pepitas and serve.

SIMPLE SWAP: You can use any hard winter squash for this recipe. Cooking time should remain about the same. If you're using acorn squash or pumpkin, cut the squash in half and scoop out the seeds, slice into crescent slices, and roast, skin-on, with the seasoning mixture. Cut the cooked squash off the skin before eating.

ROASTED ROOT VEGETABLES
WITH MEXICAN CINNAMON

SERVES 6 • PREP TIME: 20 MINUTES • COOK TIME: 1 HOUR

I once heard a chef in Mexico City say, "All you need to make anything taste Mexican is to add cinnamon." He said it in jest, but there's some truth to that. Sweet-spicy cinnamon, which was introduced into Mexican cuisine by the Spanish in the 16th century, lends itself beautifully to any Mexican dish. In this recipe, I sprinkle cinnamon on a colorful array of root vegetables for a beautifully presented, multilayered vegetable dish that's sure to please.

2 turnips, peeled, diced medium
2 rutabagas, peeled, diced medium
2 tablespoons vegetable oil, divided
2 tablespoons ground Mexican cinnamon, divided
Salt
Freshly ground black pepper

1 large sweet potato, peeled, diced medium
2 to 3 carrots, peeled, cut in ½-inch slices
2 to 3 parsnips, peeled, cut in ½-inch slices
1 large red onion, diced medium

1. Preheat the oven to 400°F.

2. In a large bowl, mix the turnips and rutabagas with 1 tablespoon of oil and 1 tablespoon of cinnamon. Season with salt and pepper.

3. Place in a large roasting pan and roast for 30 minutes.

4. In the same bowl, mix the sweet potato, carrots, parsnips, onion, and the remaining 1 tablespoon of oil and 1 tablespoon of cinnamon. Season with salt and pepper.

5. When the vegetables in the oven have cooked 30 minutes, add the sweet potato mixture to the same roasting pan. Toss the vegetables and roast for 30 minutes more, stirring about halfway through to ensure even cooking.

6. The dish is done when all the vegetables are soft but still hold their shape and have some brown to them.

SIMPLE SWAP: You can use any mix of root vegetables that you love. I encourage you to try the ones you are not a familiar with; you might find a new one to enjoy.

BAKED SWEET POTATOES
WITH BLACK BEANS, CORN, AND CHILES

MAKES 2 BAKED POTATOES • PREP TIME: 10 MINUTES • COOK TIME: 1 HOUR

Although it is hard to pin down the exact origin of the sweet potato, what we know for a fact is that the ancient Maya developed sophisticated agriculture systems to cultivate the now loved-around-the-world tuber. Packed with nutrients, sweet potatoes are the epitome of a superfood. Not only do they provide energy, but they also include a wide range of vitamins and minerals, making this the perfect base of a delicious and healthy meal.

2 large sweet potatoes, washed
2 tablespoons vegan butter
¼ cup diced white onion
2 green poblano, anaheim, or any other green chiles you like, diced small
2 garlic cloves, minced
1 cup frozen corn kernels, thawed
½ teaspoon ground cumin
½ teaspoon chili powder
1 (15-ounce) can black beans, drained and rinsed

½ teaspoon salt
½ teaspoon freshly ground black pepper
Juice of 1 lime

GARNISH OPTIONS
½ cup Aztec Spiced Pepitas (page 69)
½ cup Almond Queso Cotija (page 73)
2 teaspoons chopped cilantro

1. Poke several holes in each sweet potato using a fork—just a few pokes will be fine. Place the sweet potatoes directly on the middle rack of a cold oven, turn the heat to 425°F, and bake the potatoes for 1 hour. They are ready when a toothpick or fork inserted meets little resistance. Remove from the oven and let cool.

2. In a large skillet, heat the butter on medium-high heat. Sauté the onion, green chiles, and garlic for 5 minutes. Add the corn, cumin, and chili powder, and

cook 3 minutes more, stirring as needed. Stir in the beans and heat through. Mix in the salt, pepper, and lime juice.

3. To serve, cut open each potato lengthwise and spread it open. Top with a generous amount of the bean and corn mixture. Top with the garnishes of your choice and serve.

COOKING TIP: Why no preheating before baking the sweet potatoes? Think of it the same way you think of boiling a potato; you start with cold water for even cooking.

RICE, BEANS, AND SIDES

187

ANCHO-ROASTED SWEET POTATOES

SERVES 4 TO 6 • PREP TIME: 10 MINUTES • COOK TIME: 40 MINUTES

The state of Puebla, Mexico, boasts monumental ruins, volcanic soil, and the beloved poblano chile, star of the popular chile relleno. When dried, poblanos are called ancho chiles—heart-shaped beauties with a sweet, mild heat. Roasting sweet potatoes with ancho and onion creates a sophisticated, multilayered flavor that's simply fabulous. While there are many ways to prepare the native superfood—jam-packed with carotenoids, vitamin C, fiber, and potassium—this roasted sweet potato dish has always been a family favorite!

3 large sweet potatoes, peeled, diced medium

2 sweet yellow onions, diced medium

3 ancho chiles, rehydrated in hot water for 15 minutes, seeded, stemmed, and chopped

3 garlic cloves, minced

2 tablespoons piloncillo, crushed fine or 2 tablespoons brown sugar

1 tablespoon vegetable oil

½ teaspoon salt

½ teaspoon freshly ground black pepper

1 tablespoon vegan butter

1. Preheat the oven to 400°F.

2. In a large bowl, toss all the ingredients except the butter, and mix well with your hands.

3. Transfer to a nonstick roasting pan and roast for 30 to 40 minutes, stirring halfway through the cooking time. When the dish is done, the potatoes should still hold their shape and the onions should be nicely caramelized.

4. Remove from the oven and toss the sweet potatoes with the butter. Serve hot.

COOKING TIP: This roast reheats exceptionally well. Stuff leftovers in breakfast burritos or make roasted root vegetable tacos. Serve with your favorite vinegar hot sauce.

SAUTÉED CABBAGE WITH ONIONS, JALAPEÑOS, AND TEMPEH BACON

SERVES 4 TO 6 • PREP TIME: 10 MINUTES • COOK TIME: 20 MINUTES

However unassuming the cabbage appears, make no mistake: this cruciferous vegetable is a powerhouse! Full of vitamin C, vitamin K, folate, and fiber, cabbages are also very low-calorie. I ate cabbage all the time as a kid, whether it was in a soup or—in the case of this ranch-style recipe—as a side dish or taco topper. Sautéing cabbage with fresh onions brings out a beautiful aroma. The jalapeños deliver a little kick. And the addition of tempeh bacon is a throwback to my Norteño heritage.

1 tablespoon vegetable oil
1 white onion, julienned
1 carrot, peeled and julienned
½ cup tempeh bacon, chopped
1 to 2 jalapeño chiles, seeded and julienned
3 garlic cloves, minced
1 small head green cabbage, core removed, chopped into bite-size pieces

⅓ cup Homemade Vegetable Stock (page 231)
1 to 2 teaspoons apple cider vinegar
½ teaspoon salt
½ teaspoon freshly ground black pepper

1. In a deep, large skillet, heat the oil over medium-high heat. Add the onion, carrot, tempeh bacon, jalapeños, and garlic. Sauté for about 5 minutes. Add the cabbage and sauté for 5 minutes more.

2. Pour in the Homemade Vegetable Stock and vinegar. Bring to a boil. Reduce the heat to a simmer. Cover and simmer for 10 minutes.

3. Remove from the heat and mix in the salt and pepper. Serve warm.

COOKING TIP: If you would like to turn this into a one-pot dinner, add four of your favorite vegan sausages to the mix along with the onion. Add a large russet potato, peeled and diced small, and up the stock to 1 cup in step 2. You may have to increase the cooking time a little for the potato.

COOKING TIP: This is a 30-minute recipe if you have the vegetable stock ready made.

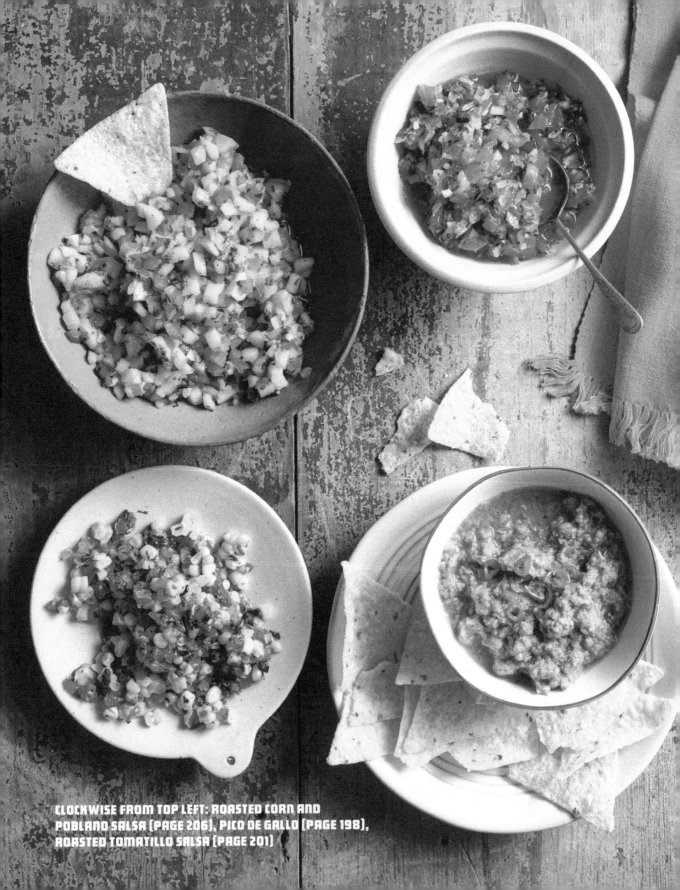

CLOCKWISE FROM TOP LEFT: ROASTED CORN AND
POBLANO SALSA (PAGE 206), PICO DE GALLO (PAGE 198),
ROASTED TOMATILLO SALSA (PAGE 201)

Chapter 8

SAUCES AND SALSAS

SPICY CHIMICHURRI

MAKES 2 CUPS • PREP TIME: 5 MINUTES, PLUS 1 HOUR CHILLING TIME

One could think of chimichurri as harnessing the flavors of the Latin American earth. The blend of seasonings—parsley, red pepper, oregano, and garlic—is unmistakably Latin. Throw in jalapeño and it's muy Mexicana! This bright, pesto-like sauce is used throughout Latin America for grilling meats, but you can use it for tofu, seitan, or anything you sling on the grill. Chimichurri sauce works wonderfully when grilling mushrooms, asparagus, and other hearty vegetables.

3 garlic cloves, minced

2 jalapeño chiles, seeded and minced

1 shallot, minced

½ bunch cilantro, thick stems removed, finely chopped

½ bunch flat-leaf parsley, thick stems removed, finely chopped

Juice of ½ lime

1 teaspoon apple cider vinegar

1 teaspoon finely chopped fresh oregano leaves

¼ teaspoon ground cumin

¼ teaspoon red chili flakes

¼ teaspoon salt, plus more for seasoning (optional)

¼ teaspoon freshly ground black pepper, plus more for seasoning (optional)

¼ cup olive oil

1. Combine all the ingredients except the olive oil in a large bowl.

2. Whisk in the oil with a fork. Season with additional salt and pepper, if needed.

3. Chill in the refrigerator at least 1 hour before serving, to let the flavors blend.

ORIGIN STORY: The word *chimichurri* comes from Basque word *tximitxurri*, which is loosely defined as "a mix of several things in no particular order." Most likely the original recipe came from Basques who had settled in Argentina.

CLASSIC CHILE PASTE

MAKES ABOUT 1 CUP • PREP TIME: 30 MINUTES • COOK TIME: 25 MINUTES

Made with spicy chiles de árbol, medium-hot guajillos, and mild anchos, this classic chile paste is the perfect condiment for bringing color and spice to any dish. I use this paste for red tamales, rice dishes, and Papas Bravas (page 82). This chile paste recipe is a milder version of the chile paste I grew up eating. To kick up the heat, simply throw in a couple more chiles de árbol. They may look small, but they pack a fiery punch!

2 dried chiles de árbol
4 dried guajillo chiles
4 dried ancho chiles

2 cups Homemade Vegetable Stock (page 231)
1 teaspoon apple cider vinegar

1. In a large bowl, steep all the chiles in hot water for 20 to 30 minutes. Drain.

2. Remove the stems and seeds, and medium dice the chiles.

3. In a large saucepan, combine the chiles, Homemade Vegetable Stock, and vinegar, and simmer for 5 to 10 minutes, or until the chiles are soft.

4. Transfer to a blender and blend until smooth.

5. Transfer back to the same saucepan and cook on medium heat, stirring constantly, for about 10 minutes or until the mixture reaches a paste-like consistency. Remove from the heat and let cool.

6. This chile paste will keep in the refrigerator for up to 7 days.

COOKING TIP: If you're in a time crunch, you can quickly reconstitute the chiles by placing them in a microwave-safe bowl, covering them with water, and microwaving for 6 minutes.

CLASSIC RED ENCHILADA SAUCE

MAKES 3 CUPS • PREP TIME: 5 MINUTES • COOK TIME: 25 MINUTES

Classic Red Enchilada Sauce should be a staple in every vegan cocina. And with this quick and easy, savory recipe, you'll never need to buy the prepackaged variety again. It starts with sautéing the onions and garlic, then lightly toasting the herbs and spices, then simmering it all with fragrant red tomatoes. Once puréed, the simple mixture transforms into a rusty red, delightfully smoky sauce. Don't limit this classic red sauce to just enchiladas. It's fantastic for smothering burritos or as a dipping sauce for chips and flautas.

1 teaspoon vegetable oil
½ white onion, diced small
1 serrano chile, seeded and minced
3 garlic cloves, minced
1 tablespoon dark chili powder or Classic Chile Paste (page 194)
2 teaspoons ground cumin
1 teaspoon dried Mexican oregano

½ teaspoon salt, plus more for seasoning (optional)
½ teaspoon freshly ground black pepper, plus more for seasoning (optional)
1 (28-ounce) can diced tomatoes, not drained
1 to 2 teaspoons apple cider vinegar

1. Heat the oil in a medium saucepan on medium-high heat. Sauté the onion, serrano chile, and garlic for 7 minutes. When the onion is soft and translucent, add the chili powder or Classic Chile Paste, cumin, oregano, salt, and pepper. Sauté for 2 minutes more.

2. Add the tomatoes and their juice, and 1 teaspoon of the vinegar. Reduce the heat to a simmer and cook, covered, for 15 minutes, stirring occasionally.

3. When the sauce has reduced to a thick, chunky sauce, transfer to a blender and purée until smooth.

4. Adjust the seasoning, adding additional teaspoons of vinegar and more salt and pepper, if needed.

COOKING TIP: This classic sauce will keep in the refrigerator for up to 7 days. Or freeze the leftovers and reheat the sauce anytime you're in the mood for Mexican flavors.

BROWN MOLE

SF

GF

MAKES 3 CUPS • PREP TIME: 20 MINUTES • COOK TIME: 30 MINUTES

*The origin story of mole sauce varies a little depending on who is telling it, but one aspect of the tale remains the same: The discovery was happenstance. Some say the cooks just took whatever ingredients were lying around the kitchen. Some say a gust of wind blew the ingredients together. This mixture (*mole *means "mix") has become a symbol of Mexico's mestizo culture; it blends earthy flavors found across the globe, including chocolate, cinnamon, and cumin, with native dried pasilla, guajillo, and ancho chiles. This classic brown mole makes a wonderfully rich topping for wet burritos and tamales, and a dipper for flautas.*

3 dried pasilla chiles
1 dried guajillo chile
1 ancho chile
2 cups water
1 tablespoon vegetable oil
2 cups white or yellow onion, diced
2 garlic cloves, minced
1 cup reserved chile liquid
1 cup Homemade Vegetable Stock
   (page 231)

5 ounces Mexican chocolate, broken up
   into small pieces
3 tablespoons smooth, unsweetened
   peanut butter
½ teaspoon ground cumin
1 corn tortilla, toasted and cut
   into pieces
Salt

1. In a large skillet, dry toast all the chiles until they are fragrant, about 5 to 7 minutes, turning once halfway through cooking. Be careful not to burn them.

2. Remove the seeds from the chiles and place the chiles in a microwave-safe bowl with the water. Microwave for 4 minutes, then let them sit in the water until they are cool to the touch.

3. In a large saucepan, heat the oil on medium-high heat. Sauté the onion and garlic until they are caramelized, about 7 minutes.

4. Transfer the mixture to a blender and add the chiles, reserved chile liquid, Homemade Vegetable Stock, Mexican chocolate, peanut butter, cumin, and tortilla pieces. Blend until smooth.

5. Transfer the mixture back to the saucepan. Bring to a boil, then simmer, covered, for 15 minutes. Use the reserved chile liquid to adjust the consistency as it simmers. Season with salt.

HEAT INDEX: When using the reserved chile liquid to adjust the consistency of this mole, just note that adding more liquid means kicking up the heat.

GREEN MOLE

MAKES 3 CUPS • PREP TIME: 15 MINUTES • COOK TIME: 30 MINUTES

Green mole is made mostly with fresh ingredients: pan-roasted fresh tomatillos, slivered onion, and spicy serrano chile, with a base of lightly toasted pepitas and cumin seeds. Mole is often made with tree nuts, and this one is nut free. Use this bright sauce to top enmoladas, tamales, burritos, or your favorite plant-based meats.

½ cup hulled pepitas
½ teaspoon whole cumin seeds
1 tablespoon vegetable oil
5 medium tomatillos, quartered (about 3 cups)
1 small white or yellow onion, sliced
4 garlic cloves, chopped

1 large serrano chile, seeded and quartered
2 cups Homemade Vegetable Stock (page 231)
½ cup chopped cilantro
1 teaspoon salt

1. In a large cast-iron skillet, dry toast the pepitas and cumin seeds for about 5 minutes or until fragrant. Transfer the toasted seeds to a food processor and process until finely ground. Or grind them with your molcajete and tejolote.

2. In the same skillet, heat the oil on medium-high heat and sauté the tomatillos, onion, garlic, and serrano chile for about 5 minutes, or until the onion is lightly browned and the tomatillos are lightly blistered.

3. Transfer the mixture to a blender. Add the Homemade Vegetable Stock, cilantro, and salt, and blend until smooth. Add the seed mix and blend until all the ingredients are well integrated.

4. Transfer back to the skillet and simmer, uncovered, for about 15 to 20 minutes. Remove from the heat.

SIMPLE SWAP: If you don't have a nut allergy, you should definitely also try this recipe with crushed peanuts in place of pumpkin seeds for a completely different flavor profile.

PICO DE GALLO

Also known as salsa fresca *or* salsa picada, *Pico de Gallo is a raw salsa made with a few simple ingredients: chopped red tomatoes, white onion, green peppers, cilantro, lime juice, and salt. This classic garnish—sometimes also called* salsa bandera *(flag sauce) in Mexico because all the colors of the Mexican flag are represented—is a great topper for anything from tacos to tortas to enchiladas, and more!*

4 large Roma tomatoes, diced
1 medium white onion, diced
2 medium serrano chiles, seeded
   and diced

2 tablespoons chopped cilantro
1 tablespoon lime juice
½ teaspoon salt

1. In a large mixing bowl, combine all the ingredients.

2. Serve fresh or chilled.

HEAT INDEX: For a milder version of this classic recipe, replace the serrano chiles with jalapeños. Jalapeños are generally three times milder than serranos.

SALSA RANCHERA

MAKES 4 CUPS • PREP TIME: 10 MINUTES • COOK TIME: 50 MINUTES

Serving as the base for my Tofu Huevos Rancheros (page 35) and as the blanket over my Classic Chile Rellenos (page 142), I bring you a Garza family Norteño-style classic: Salsa Ranchera, a spicy cooked salsa with tomatoes, serrano chiles, and a blend of herbs and spices.

2 tablespoons olive oil
½ cup diced medium green bell pepper
½ cup diced medium red bell pepper
1 to 2 serrano chiles, minced
⅓ cup diced yellow onion
3 garlic cloves, minced
1 tablespoon ground cumin
1 tablespoon chili powder
½ tablespoon dried Mexican oregano

1 (15.5-ounce) can diced tomatoes, not drained
1 (8-ounce) can tomato sauce
½ bunch fresh cilantro, chopped
1 teaspoon salt
1 teaspoon freshly ground black pepper
2 tablespoons lime juice

1. Heat the olive oil in a medium saucepan on medium-high heat. Sauté the bell peppers, serrano chiles, onion, and garlic for about 4 to 5 minutes. Add the cumin, chili powder, and oregano, and sauté for 1 to 2 minutes more.

2. Stir in the tomatoes and their juice, tomato sauce, cilantro, salt, pepper, and lime juice. Reduce the heat to a simmer. Cover and simmer for 25 to 30 minutes.

3. Remove from the heat. Cool, about 10 minutes. Blend the salsa in a blender or food processor until smooth. Serve.

ORIGIN STORY: The word *ranchera* means "ranch style," and refers to anything that fits that description, including a traditional genre of Mexican folk music that rings loud in my head every time I make this fiery sauce. Download tunes from Juan Gabriel and Rocío Dúrcal and make them part of your playlist for your next ranch-style Mexican dinner.

CHUNKY RED SALSA

MAKES 2 CUPS • PREP TIME: 5 MINUTES • COOK TIME: 30 MINUTES

I get it—we all love the popping sound of opening a brand new jar of salsa. Do yourself a favor, though, and take some time to whip up this old-school–style chunky red classic from scratch. It's outrageously simple. All you need is a large molcajete and a steady hand. And I promise, the amped-up flavors of fresh ingredients will make your taste buds sing. Serve this salsa in the molcajete; it'll be a fun conversation piece.

2 Roma tomatoes, quartered
1 garlic clove, smashed
1 tablespoon vegetable oil
1 teaspoon salt, divided, plus more for seasoning (optional)
¼ teaspoon freshly ground black pepper, plus more for seasoning (optional)
¼ teaspoon ground coriander

1 pasilla chile
1 ancho chile
2 tablespoons white onion, minced
1 chipotle chile in adobo sauce, minced
¼ cup water
Juice of 1 lime
1 tablespoon chopped cilantro

1. Preheat the oven to 425°F.

2. In a large bowl, toss the tomatoes and garlic in the oil, ½ teaspoon salt, pepper, and coriander. Transfer the tomato mix to a roasting pan and roast about 15 to 20 minutes, until browned. Remove from the oven and let it cool to the touch.

3. In a small dry skillet, toast the pasilla and ancho chiles on medium-high heat for 5 to 7 minutes, turning once. The chiles will be very fragrant when they're toasted. Cool, then seed them and break into small pieces.

4. Add ½ teaspoon salt to the molcajete and begin grinding the ingredients in this order: garlic, roasted chiles, onion, roasted tomatoes, chipotle chile. Continue grinding, adding just a little water as needed to bring the mixture together.

5. Finally, add the lime juice and the cilantro, and just stir it in. Season with additional salt and pepper, if needed.

HEAT INDEX: To turn things down, use just half of the chipotle chile.

ROASTED TOMATILLO SALSA

MAKES 3 CUPS • PREP TIME: 5 MINUTES • COOK TIME: 45 MINUTES

Tomatillos are a green fruit grown in the highlands of Guatemala, and are known as the Mexican husk tomato. Sometimes hard to find in your conventional grocery store, tomatillos can be found year-round at any Latin market. This vibrant green salsa is the perfect balance of smoky and bright to add to any dish. Made with roasted tomatillos, onion, garlic, and serrano chiles, it's especially great on my Spinach and Mushroom Enchiladas Verdes (page 148).

5 to 6 tomatillos, cut into 1½-inch
    wedges (about 3 cups)
½ cup white or yellow onion
3 garlic cloves
1 large serrano chile, seeded
1 tablespoon vegetable oil

1 cup water
2 tablespoons lime juice
2 tablespoons chopped cilantro
1 teaspoon salt
½ teaspoon freshly ground
    black pepper

1. Preheat the oven to 425°F.

2. Place the tomatillos, onion, garlic, and serrano chile in a roasting pan and toss with the oil to coat evenly. Roast for 40 to 45 minutes, or until the onion is nicely toasted but not burned.

3. Transfer the roasted tomatillos and veggies, water, lime juice, cilantro, salt, and pepper to a blender, and blend until there are no large chunks.

4. Serve warm or cold.

SECRET INGREDIENT: Because tomatillos are naturally high in pectin, this home-made salsa will thicken and gel after refrigerating. To loosen it up, simply stir with a fork.

AVOCADO TOMATILLO SALSA

MAKES 2½ TO 3 CUPS • PREP TIME: 10 MINUTES

The tomatillo, also known as the Mexican husk tomato or tomate in Mexico, is the cousin to the better-known red tomato in the US. Neatly wrapped in a thin, papery skin is how you'll typically find this plump green nightshade. In this salsa, tangy tomatillos mingle with rich, creamy avocados to create a show-stopping salsa that deserves a place in every cook's repertoire. Add a little variety to your kitchen with this happy, bright-green salsa. It's guaranteed to liven up any table or dish.

5 fresh tomatillos, quartered
¼ white onion, roughly chopped
1 to 3 serrano chiles, seeded and
    roughly chopped
2 garlic cloves, roughly chopped
¼ cup water
2 small or 1 large avocado, peeled
    and pitted

Juice of 1 lime
¼ teaspoon ground coriander
¼ teaspoon salt
¼ teaspoon freshly ground
    black pepper
2 tablespoons chopped cilantro

1. Put the tomatillos, onion, serranos, and garlic in the blender with a splash of water to get the blender moving. Blend to a chunky texture.

2. Add the avocados, lime juice, coriander, salt, and pepper, and blend until it is as smooth as you desire. Add the cilantro and pulse until just blended.

3. This salsa will keep in the refrigerator for about 1 week.

HEAT INDEX: Adjust the heat by varying the number of serrano chiles in this recipe. One serrano will make a mild salsa; two will be medium to medium-hot; three will be hot to burning hot.

CHILES DE ÁRBOL SALSA

SF

GF

NF

Q&E

MAKES 2 CUPS • PREP TIME: 5 MINUTES • COOK TIME: 10 MINUTES

Warning: This fiery sauce is no joke. It's muy picante! The heat of one single chile de árbol goes a long way—and this sauce calls for 10 of them. Chile de árbol, which means "tree chile," refers to the chile plant's size—it's large enough to be considered a small tree. The spicy chile is also some-times called pico de pajara *(bird beak chile) and* cola de rata *(rat tail chile) because of its slender, long shape. Use this salsa when you really want to add heat to your dish!*

2 tablespoons olive oil
10 dried chiles de árbol, seeded
   (save the seeds)
2 dried pasilla chiles, seeded
½ white onion, diced medium
2 garlic cloves, smashed

3 Roma tomatoes, quartered
1 tablespoon apple cider vinegar
¼ teaspoon salt
¼ teaspoon freshly ground
   black pepper
1 teaspoon toasted sesame seeds

1. In a medium saucepan, heat the oil on medium heat and fry the chiles for about 5 minutes. Do not burn the chiles or they will become bitter. Remove the chiles from the pan.

2. Sauté the onion and garlic in the same pan for about 7 minutes, then add the tomatoes and sauté 3 minutes more.

3. Transfer the mixture to a blender, add the cooked chiles and the reserved chiles de árbol seeds, vinegar, salt, and pepper. Purée until smooth.

4. Serve in a bowl garnished with toasted sesame seeds.

HEAT INDEX: The reserved seeds will make the salsa even hotter, so you can leave them out if it's already plenty hot. Chiles de árbol are pretty easy to find. If you can't find them in your area, japones, pequin, and tepin chiles are all excellent substitutes.

MANGO SALSA

SF

GF

NF

MAKES 2 CUPS • PREP TIME: 10 MINUTES, PLUS 1 HOUR CHILLING TIME

When mouthwatering mango comes into season, you can find me at the farmers' market buying 10 at a time. Mango salsa is a great way to bring more sweetness into your life too, and this recipe provides a refreshing twist on the classic salsa that many of us have come to know and love. For this tropical salsa, mango is combined with the crunchy kick of red onion and the heat of serrano chiles.

2 large or 4 small mangos, peeled and
    diced small
2 serrano chiles, seeded and minced
½ red onion, diced small
1 red bell pepper, seeded and
    diced small

2 tablespoons chopped cilantro
Juice of ½ lime
¼ teaspoon salt
¼ teaspoon freshly ground
    black pepper

1. Mix all ingredients in a large bowl and refrigerate for at least 1 hour.

2. This salsa will keep well in the refrigerator for 3 to 4 days.

SECRET INGREDIENT: This is a very simple version of tropical mango salsa. Adding in some other tropical fruits, such as pineapple or ripe papaya, will elevate your salsa to another level. Also, try all kinds of mangoes for this recipe: Ataulfos, Kent, Haden, and Keitt. Each variety has something different to offer.

RED ONION, RADISH, AND CILANTRO RELISH

MAKES 2 CUPS • PREP TIME: 10 MINUTES, PLUS 1 HOUR CHILLING TIME

Sometimes it's the simplest things. And this relish is one of those things for me. At home, I call this "the everything garnish," because it's a perfect topper for everything. This simple combination of julienned red onion and radish, tossed with cilantro, fresh lime juice, and just a dash of salt and pepper is the perfect topper for tacos, fajitas, sopes, and everything in between.

1 bunch red radishes (at least 10), greens removed, julienned
1 small red onion, cut in half and julienned
Juice of ¼ lime
¼ bunch chopped cilantro
½ teaspoon salt
½ teaspoon freshly ground black pepper

1. Mix all the ingredients in a large bowl.

2. Cover and refrigerate at least 1 hour before serving.

COOKING TIP: You can store this relish in a covered container in the refrigerator for up to 1 week. The flavor and color will intensify (for the better, in my opinion).

ROASTED CORN AND POBLANO SALSA

MAKES 2 CUPS • PREP TIME: 10 MINUTES • COOK TIME: 20 MINUTES, PLUS 1 HOUR CHILLING TIME

Made popular by American burrito chains as a burrito stuffing or topping for burrito bowls, corn salsas have built a strong fan base throughout the US and even some parts of Mexico. For this corn salsa recipe, I combine the smoky flavors of a roasted poblano chile with roasted fresh shucked corn, which brings out its naturally sweet, slightly nutty flavors. Roasted alongside fragrant jalapeño and ripe Roma tomatoes, this hearty salsa offers a delightful accent to Tex-Mex classics.

Kernels from 4 ears fresh corn or
   3 cups frozen corn kernels, thawed
½ red onion, diced small
1 jalapeño chile, seeded and
   diced small
½ teaspoon ground cumin
½ teaspoon salt, plus more
   for seasoning

½ teaspoon freshly ground black
   pepper, plus more for seasoning
1 poblano chile, charred, skinned,
   seeded, and diced small
4 Roma tomatoes, diced small
3 tablespoons chopped cilantro
1 tablespoon vegetable oil
Juice of 1 lime

1. Preheat the oven to 400°F.

2. In a medium bowl, mix the corn, onion, jalapeño, cumin, salt, and pepper. Transfer to a roasting pan. Roast for 20 minutes, stirring halfway through the cooking time. Remove from the oven and set aside to cool.

3. In the same bowl, mix the charred poblano chile, tomatoes, cilantro, and oil. Add the roasted vegetables. Season with salt and pepper, and add the lime juice.

4. Refrigerate for 1 hour, and serve cold. This salsa will keep for up to 1 week in the refrigerator.

COOKING TIP: To roast the poblano, lightly oil and place the chile in the oven at 425°F for about 10 minutes, turning halfway through the cooking time. When the chile is blistered all over, remove from the oven and place in a bowl. Cover with plastic wrap. Set aside to cool, so the skin will be easy to remove.

ROASTED CHAYOTE AND JALAPEÑO SALSA

MAKES 2 CUPS • PREP TIME: 10 MINUTES • COOK TIME: 20 MINUTES

Chayote squash, native to Mesoamerica, is a super healthy food that is a very good source of fiber, vitamin C, zinc, and potassium. When the Spanish came to Mexico, they brought with them a lot of new crops and culinary methods, but what they also did was take back to Europe many crops that were new to them too. The chayote is a stellar example of this exchange, and now this crop is found everywhere from Europe to Thailand to Australia. This salsa is just one great way to use this super squash!

1 chayote, peeled, diced small
½ red onion, diced small
1 jalapeño chile, seeded and minced
3 red sweet mini peppers, seeded and
    diced small, or ¼ cup diced and
    seeded red bell peppers
1 garlic clove, minced
½ teaspoon ground cumin

1 tablespoon vegetable oil, divided
Salt
Freshly ground black pepper
6 Roma tomatoes, quartered
Juice of 1 lime
2 tablespoons chopped cilantro
Whole cilantro leaves
1 teaspoon toasted sesame seeds

1. Preheat the oven to 425°F.

2. In a large bowl, toss the chayote, onion, jalapeño, peppers, garlic, and cumin with ½ tablespoon oil. Season with salt and pepper.

3. In a separate bowl, toss the tomatoes with ½ tablespoon oil and season with salt and pepper.

4. Place the veggies from each bowl onto two separate roasting pans.

5. Roast all the veggies for 20 minutes, stirring halfway through the cooking time.

6. Mash the roasted tomatoes in a molcajete to achieve a slightly chunky consistency.

7. Fold the rest of the ingredients from the other roasting pan, along with the lime juice and chopped cilantro, into the mashed tomatoes.

8. Serve warm in a bowl, topped with cilantro leaves and toasted sesame seeds.

COOKING TIP: This also works as a cold salsa. You can keep it in an airtight container in your refrigerator for up to 1 week.

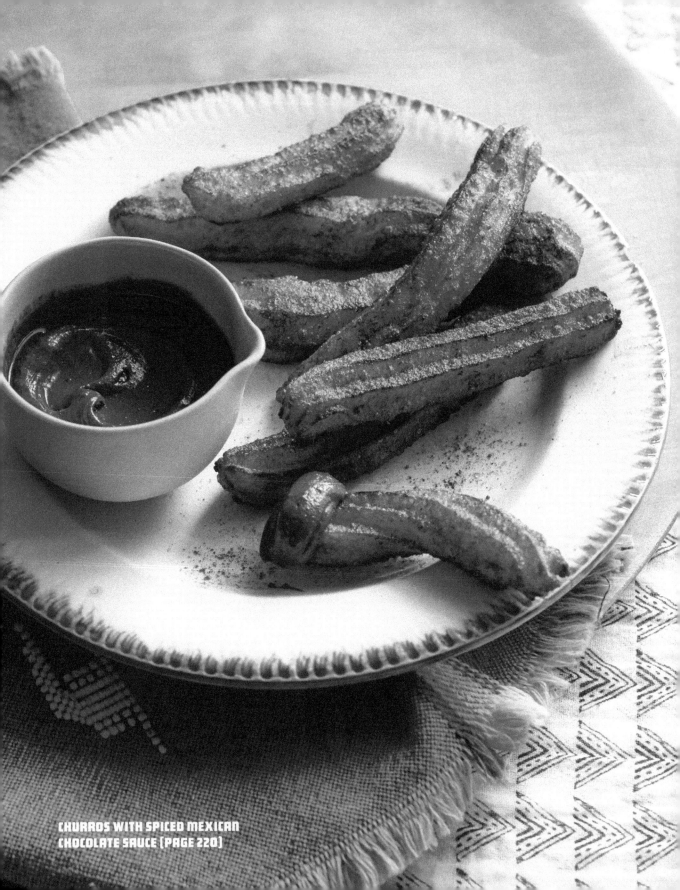

CHURROS WITH SPICED MEXICAN
CHOCOLATE SAUCE (PAGE 220)

Chapter 9

DRINKS AND DESSERTS

CAFÉ SIN LECHE

SERVES 4 • PREP TIME: 2 MINUTES • COOK TIME: 10 MINUTES

Although coffee is not native to Mexico, the country is now one of the largest coffee producers in the world. Coffee first arrived in Mexico in the late 1700s, when the Spanish entered the port of Veracruz with coffee plants from the Caribbean islands. The state of Veracruz is the second largest producer of coffee in Mexico. It's largely grown in the mountainous regions of Xalapa, Coatepec, and Orizaba for use in candies, baked goods, and, of course, for drinking. In the city of Veracruz is a centuries-old café called Gran Café de La Parroquia, which is world-renowned for its Spanish influenced café con leche (coffee with milk). Here, I bring you a dairy-free rendition of the classic coffee drink to enjoy with all your favorite Mexican breakfasts and desserts.

3 cups water
4 tablespoons ground coffee

3 cups unsweetened almond milk
Sugar

1. Bring the water to a boil.

2. Add the ground coffee to a French press coffeemaker. Pour the boiling water over the coffee and put the lid on. Steep for 5 to 7 minutes.

3. While the coffee is steeping, heat the almond milk in a small saucepan on medium-high heat until it just boils. Remove from the heat.

4. By this point, the coffee should be ready to press, so use the plunger to press the coffee down.

5. To serve, pour the coffee into 4 cups, then pour the scalded almond milk into each cup. You'll have equal amounts coffee and almond milk.

6. Sweeten as desired.

COOKING TIP: If you don't have a French press, use your favorite drip coffeemaker or espresso machine to brew coffee at your preferred strength. Serve with equal portions of unsweetened almond milk.

CHAMPURRADO

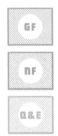

SERVES 8 • PREP TIME: 5 MINUTES • COOK TIME: 20 MINUTES

Champurrado is a kind of atole—*a traditional beverage made by toasting masa on a griddle, then adding water that was boiled with cinnamon sticks. The resulting atole can be thick or thin, depending on how it's made. Champurrado is ancient Mexican hot chocolate; it dates back the 14th century, and it's as popular today as it was back then. In fact, you'll even find champurrado served Frappuccino-style in certain hip parts of Mexico these days. At Casa Garza, I always make this classic chocolate-based drink on Christmas Eve and New Year's. Enjoy this comforting, celebratory beverage with Churros (page 220) or your favorite tamales. Be careful not to burn yourself serving and drinking champurrado. Because it's so thick, it gets really hot and maintains heat longer than regular hot chocolate.*

4 cups soy milk
2½ cups water
1 large cinnamon stick
1 (8-ounce) cone piloncillo, broken into small pieces

5½ ounces Mexican chocolate, broken into pieces
½ cup corn masa flour

1. In large pot, bring the soy milk, water, cinnamon stick, piloncillo, and chocolate to a boil. Lower the heat and simmer until the piloncillo and chocolate have dissolved, about 7 to 10 minutes. Stir constantly.

2. Add the corn masa flour, a little at a time, using a whisk to stir constantly until the drink has thickened to a gravy-like consistency.

3. Serve immediately.

ORIGIN STORY: Corn masa flour is made from nixtimalized and ground maize, and is not the regular cornmeal you find at the supermarket. You can get it at any Latin grocery or well-stocked supermarket. My favorite brand is Maseca.

HORCHATA MEXICANA

SF

GF

NF

MAKES ABOUT 4 CUPS • PREP TIME: 5 MINUTES, PLUS 3 HOURS SOAKING TIME • COOK TIME: 7 MINUTES

Mexican horchata is a delightful beverage made with rice, cinnamon, sugar, and Mexican vanilla, and is typically served chilled. Often, you'll find this drink sold alongside other aguas frescas *("fresh waters"). For this classic Mexican horchata recipe, I lightly brown the rice and cinnamon sticks to bring out their wonderful nuttiness, making the end result an aromatic and earthy refreshment that is unmistakably* Mexicana!

½ cup white rice
2 cinnamon sticks
2 cups water
¼ to ½ cup sugar, dissolved in ½ cup warm water

1 teaspoon Mexican vanilla extract
¼ teaspoon salt
2 cups rice milk
Cinnamon sticks and ground cinnamon, for garnish

1. In a skillet on medium heat, dry sauté the rice and cinnamon sticks for about 5 to 7 minutes, or until the rice begins to lightly brown.

2. Add the rice and cinnamon sticks to a blender and blend on high for 1 minute, so they are broken down into a coarse powder.

3. Pour in the water and let the rice-cinnamon mixture sit for at least 3 hours or overnight in the refrigerator.

4. Strain through a fine mesh strainer or a doubled layer of cheesecloth into a pitcher or large bowl. You may want to strain it twice to get as much of the rice grit as possible out of the liquid.

5. Add the sugar syrup, vanilla, salt, and rice milk to the cinnamon rice water and whisk until the sugar syrup is dissolved.

6. Serve well chilled over ice, with a cinnamon stick and some ground cinnamon on top.

SIMPLE SWAP: There are many regional variations on Horchata—too many to list! Some add blanched almonds or peanuts to the mix in the soaking and blending stages. I've even had it with sesame seeds.

CAPIROTADA

SERVES 12 • PREP TIME: 30 MINUTES • COOK TIME: 55 MINUTES

Capirotada is Mexican bread pudding traditionally served during the Lenten season. There are many ways to prepare it, but the base ingredients are always the same and are richly symbolic of the Passion in Christianity. The bread represents the body of Jesus, the syrup represents his blood, the cloves—clavo in Spanish, which means both "clove" and "nail"—represent the nails used for the crucifixion, and the cinnamon sticks represent the wood of the cross. For me and my family during childhood, capirotada was an essential dish on Good Friday—though you can enjoy this delicious bread pudding year-round.

8 ounces piloncillo
2 cinnamon sticks
4 whole cloves
¼ teaspoon Mexican vanilla extract
4 cups water

4 medium-large bolillos
½ cup vegan butter
¾ cup raisins
¾ cup chopped walnuts
1 cup mild vegan shredded cheese

1. In a large pot, combine the piloncillo, cinnamon, cloves, vanilla, and water and bring to a boil. Remove from the heat and let steep until the piloncillo is fully dissolved.

2. Preheat the oven to 350°F.

3. Slice the bolillos into 1-inch slices. Butter the slices on both sides and lay flat on one or two large baking sheets. Toast the bread in the oven for 4 to 5 minutes on each side.

4. Use a strainer to remove the cinnamon sticks and cloves from the sugar syrup. Measure 1½ cups of liquid.

5. In a large, deep casserole, place a layer of toasted bread slices, packed as tightly as possible. Top the layer with ¼ cup of raisins, ¼ cup of walnuts, and ⅓ cup of cheese. Pour 1 cup of syrup all over the layer. Allow about 5 minutes for the bread to soak up all the syrup. Repeat with two more layers, ending with a layer of cheese.

6. Cover the dish with aluminum foil and bake for 45 minutes. Uncover and bake for 10 minutes more, or until the top layer of cheese is completely melted. Serve hot.

SECRET INGREDIENT: While cheese might seem an unlikely ingredient for dessert, it's important in this dish because it symbolizes the shroud used to bury Jesus. I use Follow Your Heart brand shreds for this recipe because it has a nice mild taste that works well with this sweet bread pudding.

CINNAMON-RAISIN TAMALES

SF

GF

NF

MAKES 12 TAMALES • PREP TIME: 15 MINUTES, PLUS 1 HOUR SOAKING TIME •
COOK TIME: 35 TO 40 MINUTES, PLUS 15 MINUTES RESTING TIME

*When I was a kid, one of the best parts about Christmas morning was
waking up to the smell of tamales steaming on the stovetop. Grandma
always had a few pots going, and I always looked forward to the
torpedo-shaped tamales because I knew they were the sweet ones. These
subtly sweet and delicately spiced cinnamon-raisin tamales were—
and remain—a Garza family favorite. Enjoy these with a hot cup of
Champurrado (page 212) or Café sin Leche (page 211).*

1 (8-ounce) package dried corn husks
3 cups corn masa flour
1 teaspoon baking powder
4 tablespoons sugar
1 teaspoon ground cinnamon

⅛ teaspoon ground cloves
5 tablespoons vegetable shortening
2¾ cups warm water
¼ cup raisins

1. TO PREPARE THE CORN HUSKS: In a large pot, submerge the corn husks in hot water for 1 hour to make them pliable.

2. When the husks are pliable, select about 20 of the largest and most flexible. Make sure all the selected husks have no holes in them. Pat dry and set aside 12 of them.

3. Tear the remaining 18 husks into twenty-four ½-inch strips for tying.

1. TO MAKE THE BATTER: In a large bowl, whisk together the masa flour, baking powder, sugar, cinnamon, and cloves.

2. Add the shortening and use your hands to combine. Add the water and mix well. The consistency should be thicker than pancake batter, but not as thick as cookie batter. It should be spreadable using the back of a spoon.

3. Fold in the raisins and combine.

1. TO MAKE THE TAMALES: Place about 4 tablespoons of batter in the center of a corn husk. Gently roll the husk over to surround the filling. Tie both ends with corn husk strips. Repeat until all 12 tamales are formed.

2. Put about 2 inches of water in a large, deep steaming pot. Add a steamer basket, making sure the water line is below the basket. Place the tamales upright in the basket. Cover and steam for about 35 to 40 minutes, adding more water to the pot as needed. Remove from the heat.

3. Let the tamales sit, uncovered, in the pot for about 15 minutes, or until they are firm and pull away from husk easily.

4. Serve the tamales warm.

BUÑUELOS WITH CINNAMON PILONCILLO AND CARAMEL SAUCE

MAKES 8 BUÑUELOS • PREP TIME: 5 MINUTES • COOK TIME: 25 MINUTES

Every year around Christmas, my family would eat these sweet and cinnamon-y deep-fried crispy tortillas. I remember hovering outside my grandmother's kitchen with my brother and cousins, waiting eagerly for the first hot stack of buñuelos to come out. When we were kids, we would just dig right in. For this recipe, we are going to add a fun caramel dip to ramp things up. These go over best served at any winter holiday party, alongside a hot cup of Champurrado (page 212).

FOR THE CARAMEL SAUCE
1¼ cups unsweetened almond milk, divided
½ cup small piloncillo pieces
¼ cup sugar
½ teaspoon Mexican vanilla extract
Pinch of salt
½ teaspoon ground cinnamon
2 tablespoons vegan butter
1 tablespoon cornstarch or arrowroot powder

FOR THE BUÑUELOS
½ cup sugar
4 tablespoons ground cinnamon
¼ cup vegetable oil
8 Handmade Flour Tortillas (page 233), pressed but uncooked

1. TO MAKE THE CARAMEL SAUCE: In a medium saucepan, bring 1 cup almond milk, piloncillo, sugar, and vanilla to a boil. Reduce the heat and simmer 10 to 15 minutes, whisking frequently to prevent the sugar from burning.

2. Once the sugars have caramelized and the mixture has reduced a bit, lower the heat to medium.

3. Add the salt and cinnamon and stir to combine. Then whisk in the butter.

4. In a small bowl, whisk together ¼ cup cold almond milk and the cornstarch. Add to the saucepan, whisking constantly to prevent lumps.

5. Bring the mixture to a simmer and cook for about 5 minutes, until the sauce is thick and very smooth.

6. Remove from the heat. Set aside and keep warm.

7. This sauce will keep in the refrigerator for 1 week.

1. **TO MAKE THE BUÑUELOS:** Mix the sugar and cinnamon and spread evenly across a plate large enough to drop a tortilla on.

2. Heat the oil in a deep, large skillet on medium-high heat. Carefully fry each tortilla about 15 to 20 seconds on each side, or until it is brown and slightly crisp. If large bubbles develop, you can either leave them be or poke a small hole in them with a fork or toothpick. Remove each tortilla from the oil, and briefly drain it on a rack over a baking sheet or on paper towels.

3. Coat each warm buñuelo by dropping it onto the cinnamon and sugar plate, then flip to coat the other side.

4. Stack the coated buñuelos on a paper towel-lined plate.

5. To serve, place the buñuelo stack on a plate next to a bowl filled with the caramel sauce, and make sure it is within arm's reach of your eager loved ones.

COOKING TIP: For best results, roll out each tortilla and stack them on a large dinner plate between pieces of waxed paper. Wrap the dinner plate and tortilla stack in plastic wrap and place in the refrigerator. Chill the raw tortillas for about 1 hour before frying.

MEXICAN CHOCOLATE CAKE

MAKES 1 THREE-LAYER CAKE OR 30 CUPCAKES • PREP TIME: 20 MINUTES
COOK TIME: 30 MINUTES

Perfect for any quinceañera or birthday celebration—or just a Tuesday night indulgence—this perfectly balanced three-layer cake carries the traditional sweet flavors of Mexico in every luscious morsel.

FOR THE CAKE
2⅔ cups all-purpose flour (12 ounces)
⅜ cup natural cocoa powder (not Dutch) (1.3 ounces)
2 teaspoons ground cinnamon
1 teaspoon baking soda
½ teaspoon salt
2 cups sugar (14 ounces)
½ cup vegetable oil (4 ounces)
1 cup vegan mayo (8 ounces)
1½ cups hot water (12 ounces)
1 teaspoon white vinegar

FOR THE ICING
1½ cups vegan butter (12 ounces)
1 cup cocoa powder
8 tablespoons corn syrup
7½ cups powdered sugar (2 pounds)
2 tablespoons unsweetened almond milk

1. TO MAKE THE CAKE: Preheat the oven to 350°F. Lightly grease three 8-inch round baking pans or enough cupcake tins for 30 cupcakes.

2. In a large bowl, mix the flour, cocoa powder, cinnamon, baking soda, and salt. Set aside.

3. Using an electric mixer or a hand beater, beat together the sugar, vegetable oil, and mayo until creamy. Add the flour mixture and continue beating.

4. Add the hot water and beat for 2 to 3 minutes. Add the vinegar and beat for another 1 to 2 minutes.

5. Evenly fill the cake pans or cupcake tin. Bake for 20 minutes. When the cake is done, it should be springy in the center when touched, and a toothpick inserted in the center will come out clean.

1. TO MAKE THE ICING: In a large bowl, mix the butter, cocoa powder, and corn syrup into a paste. Add all the powdered sugar, and beat on low speed using an electric mixer (or use a hand beater), until everything is well combined.

2. Add the almond milk, 1 teaspoon at a time, beating between each one, until the icing is creamy. Be careful that it does not become too soft.

1. **TO ICE THE CAKE:** Let the cake cool completely on a wire rack before icing it.

2. Cut the tops off each cake to make them level. Spread a coating of icing onto the top of two cake layers, then stack all three layers. Spread a coating of icing over the top and sides of the cake.

3. Alternately, frost the top of each cupcake.

4. Decorate the cake or cupcakes with powdered sugar and cinnamon, and serve with fresh raspberries.

SECRET INGREDIENT: Vegan cakes are very unforgiving, and mine did not turn out well for years. I finally ended up working in a bakery, where I learned the secret of making perfect vegan cakes: You have to weigh the ingredients. I've given you the weights and strongly urge you to use a digital scale to weigh everything; the results will be worth it.

CHURROS WITH SPICED MEXICAN CHOCOLATE SAUCE

MAKES ABOUT 20 CHURROS • PREP TIME: 10 MINUTES, PLUS 20 MINUTES CHILLING TIME • COOK TIME: 30 MINUTES

Churros are great for breakfast or any time. And they pair perfectly with a nice Café sin Leche (page 211). Often considered an early-morning to late-morning street food, it also makes sense to place churros into the same family as doughnuts and crullers. Whether churros were invented by the Spanish, Portuguese, or Chinese (all three claim it), we can all agree: They are delicious. Even so, let's take things to another level here by dipping them in Mexican spiced chocolate sauce.

FOR THE CHURROS
2 cups water
1 cup sugar, plus 2 tablespoons
½ teaspoon salt
½ teaspoon Mexican vanilla extract
4 cups vegetable oil, divided
2 cups all-purpose flour
4 tablespoons ground cinnamon

FOR THE SAUCE
1 cup full-fat unsweetened coconut milk
½ cup unsweetened almond milk
1 cup semisweet vegan chocolate chips
6 ounces Mexican chocolate, roughly chopped or broken into small pieces
½ teaspoon cayenne pepper, or to taste
Pinch of salt

1. TO MAKE THE CHURROS: In a medium saucepan on medium heat, combine the water, 1 cup of sugar, salt, vanilla, and 2 tablespoons of oil. Bring to a boil, then promptly remove from the heat.

2. Add the flour and stir with a sturdy wooden spoon, making sure all the flour is completely mixed in. Check to make sure there are no pockets of dry flour hiding in your dough.

3. Allow the dough to cool for a few minutes, then place it into a cloth piping bag with a large star tip on it. The large tip ensures you are not working too hard to squeeze the dough out.

4. Pipe out your churros, about 4 inches long, onto a nonstick or wax paper–lined baking sheet, and refrigerate for 20 minutes. Cold churro dough is easy to handle and fries better.

5. In a large pot, bring the rest of the vegetable oil to 350°F, using a thermometer to keep an eye on the oil temperature. This is very important for getting a nicely fried churro. You may have to adjust the heat on your stovetop to keep the oil at a constant temperature during frying.

6. Slide a few churros into the oil. Make sure to leave enough room for them to float around in the pot. Fry the churros until they are golden brown, about 3 to 4 minutes each.

7. Remove the churros from the oil with a slotted spoon or tongs. Let them drain on a rack over a baking sheet or on paper towels.

8. Combine the remaining 2 tablespoons of sugar with the cinnamon in a large bowl. Toss the churros around in the bowl, a few at a time, to coat.

9. Serve drizzled with Mexican Spiced Chocolate Sauce.

1. TO MAKE THE SAUCE: Bring the coconut milk and almond milk to a boil over medium-high heat, then promptly remove from the heat.

2. Whisk the chocolate chips and pieces of Mexican chocolate a little at a time into the hot milks, until everything is melted and combined.

3. Stir in the cayenne and salt.

4. Keep warm on the stovetop next to the heat but not on a direct flame.

COOKING TIP: The churro dough will keep in the piping bag for a couple of days in the refrigerator if you aren't making them all at once.

CONCHAS

MAKES 8 CONCHAS • PREP TIME: 20 MINUTES, PLUS 1 HOUR RISING TIME • COOK TIME: 25 MINUTES

If I had to name my favorite Mexican sweet bread when I was growing up, it would hands down be the concha. From a very early age, I remember relishing freshly baked conchas before they even had a chance to cool. After I went vegan, though, I had a hard time finding conchas made without dairy or eggs. Thankfully, my baking days at Spiral Diner & Bakery in Dallas taught me that you can bake delicious dairy- and egg-free versions of virtually any yeast bread. Named for its seashell pattern topping, conchas are made up of two parts: the lightly sweetened yeast dough base, and the crumbly cookie topping. Enjoy one (or two—or three!) with a warm cup of Café sin Leche (page 211).

FOR THE CONCHAS
⅔ cup warm unsweetened almond milk
⅓ cup warm water
3 teaspoons dry active yeast
2 tablespoons sugar, divided
3 cups all-purpose flour, divided
⅓ cup plus 2 tablespoons
   vegan butter
1 teaspoon salt

FOR THE TOPPING
¼ cup sugar
¼ cup vegan butter
⅓ cup all-purpose flour
¼ teaspoon ground cinnamon
¼ teaspoon vanilla extract
6 drops of food coloring
   of your choice (optional)

1. **TO MAKE THE CONCHAS:** Pour the warm almond milk and water in a large bowl. Sprinkle the yeast over the mixture and add 1 tablespoon of sugar. Whisk and set aside until the mixture foams, about 5 to 6 minutes.

2. Add 2 cups of flour, the remaining 1 tablespoon of sugar, and the butter to the yeast mixture. Using a dough hook on a standing mixer, mix for 2 to 3 minutes. Add the remaining 1 cup of flour and the salt. Mix for 8 more minutes or until the dough is soft and smooth.

3. If you don't have a standing mixer, use a dough spatula to scrape flour from the edges and knead with hands to squish away any dry spots to fully incorporate dough.

4. Place the dough in a lightly oiled bowl. Cover the bowl with a towel and set in a warm area to double in size, about 1 to 2 hours.

5. While the dough is rising, make the topping and preheat the oven to 350°F. Lightly grease one or two baking sheets.

6. When dough has doubled, punch it down and let it rest for 10 minutes.

7. Divide the dough into 8 balls. Place each ball on the greased baking sheet. Place a disc of topping on each ball. Using a sharp paring knife, cut a shell pattern on each.

8. Bake for 25 minutes. Serve hot.

1. **TO MAKE THE TOPPING:** Beat the sugar and butter together with an electric mixer or by hand.

2. Stir in the flour, cinnamon, vanilla, and food coloring (if using).

3. Form into 8 balls, and roll each out into a disc on a lightly floured surface. Set aside.

COOKING TIP: Conchas are best eaten right out of the oven, but they'll keep well for up to 2 days in an airtight container. To reheat, simply wrap the concha in a paper towel and microwave for 15 to 20 seconds.

SPICED PUMPKIN EMPANADAS

MAKES 12 SMALL EMPANADAS • PREP TIME: 15 MINUTES, PLUS 4 HOURS
CHILLING TIME • COOK TIME: 20 MINUTES, PLUS 10 MINUTES RESTING TIME

*Looking for a warm, rich dessert for your fall festivities? Look no further.
This classic empanada, easily made vegan by using dairy-free cream
cheese, is sure to impress guests at all your autumn feasts. This sweet
pumpkin empanada is a spiced-up version of the kind you'll most often
find at Mexican bakeries in my Tex-Mex border hometown of Brownsville.
The dough rolls better if it's cold, so if you have the time, let it rest in the
refrigerator overnight, wrapped in plastic wrap. Garnish the finished
empanadas with a sprinkle of powdered sugar and cinnamon, and enjoy.*

FOR THE FILLING
1 (15-ounce) can pumpkin purée
1 (8-ounce) cone piloncillo, broken
    into pieces
1 tablespoon ground cinnamon
¼ teaspoon ground nutmeg

FOR THE EMPANADAS
1 (8-ounce) package vegan
    cream cheese
½ cup vegan butter
1¾ cups all-purpose flour

1. TO MAKE THE FILLING: Place all the ingredients in a medium saucepan over low heat. Cook until the piloncillo is completely melted.

2. Chill at least 4 hours in the refrigerator.

1. TO MAKE THE EMPANADAS: Mix all the ingredients in a large bowl until they are well-combined. Chill the dough for 3 hours.

2. Preheat the oven to 375°F.

3. Divide the dough into 12 small balls and roll out to round discs, about 5 inches in diameter.

4. Spoon 2 to 2½ tablespoons of filling onto the center of each disc. Fold the dough over, lightly wet the edges, and press together to seal. Press fork along sealed edges to lock in the seal.

5. Place the empanadas on a baking sheet and bake 15 to 20 minutes, or until it is golden brown.

6. Let the empanadas sit for 10 minutes before serving. Serve warm or cold.

ORIGIN STORY: Empanadas are stuffed bread or pastry that are baked or fried. The name comes from the Spanish word *empanar*—meaning "to coat with bread." Empanadas trace their origins to Galicia, in the northwest region of Spain, and are one of Spain's most beloved contributions to Latin cuisine. A Spanish cookbook published in 1520 mentions seafood empanadas.

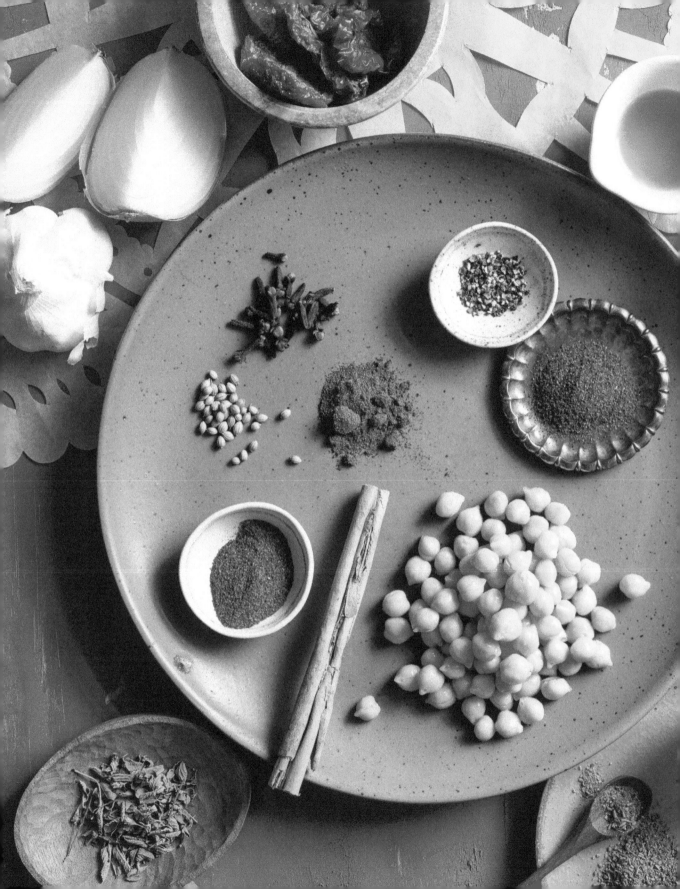

Chapter 10

STAPLES

AZTEC SPICE BLEND

MAKES ABOUT ¼ CUP • PREP TIME: 5 MINUTES

This spice blend combines earthy ancho chile and smoky chipotle with garlic, cumin, and cinnamon to season all your favorite plant-based meats. When cooking with this blend, especially when you are searing, make sure there is plenty of ventilation. This smoke from this spicy combination can get pretty intense when cooking in small spaces like my tiny loft apartment.

2 teaspoons salt
1 teaspoon garlic powder
2 teaspoons ground cumin
2 teaspoons chipotle powder
½ teaspoon ancho chili powder

1 teaspoon freshly ground black pepper
½ teaspoon ground cinnamon
2 teaspoons dried Mexican oregano
1 teaspoon dried thyme

1. In a small bowl, combine all the ingredients.

2. Store in an airtight container in your spice cabinet for up to 30 days.

ORIGIN STORY: The ancient Aztecs used a wide variety of native plants to season foods. The most important were chiles, which were often roasted, dried, and ground to be incorporated into dishes. Spanish conquistadores introduced the Aztecs to a whole new world of aromatic spices, which they merged with chiles to create the modern Mexican flavors we know and love today.

CASHEW CREMA MEXICANA

MAKES 4 CUPS • PREP TIME: 15 MINUTES

Nothing complements fiery dishes like this cool and refreshing Cashew Crema Mexicana. This dairy-free version of the popular Mexican condiment is perfect for balancing the heat of spicy enchiladas, enmoladas, chile rellenos, and more. Brightened with fresh lime juice and just a splash of apple cider vinegar, this versatile cream sauce can serve as a wonderful base for creamy salad dressing or as a substitute for sour cream or fresh cream.

2 cups raw cashew pieces
1 cup water
Juice of 2 limes

1 teaspoon salt
1 teaspoon apple cider vinegar

1. Place the cashews in a microwave-safe bowl and add enough water to cover. Microwave on high for 6 to 8 minutes, then let soak for an additional 10 minutes.

2. Alternatively, you can soak the cashews for 12 to 24 hours in the refrigerator.

3. Drain and rinse the cashews with cold water.

4. Place in a blender with at least 1 cup of water and blend on high until very smooth, adding a little bit of water at a time to adjust the consistency.

5. Add the lime juice, salt, and vinegar. Blend for 1 minute more. Adjust the seasonings.

COOKING TIP: This multiuse condiment stores very well. Keep it in the refrigerator in an airtight container for up to 1 week.

HOMEMADE VEGETABLE STOCK

MAKES 1 GALLON • PREP TIME: 5 MINUTES • COOK TIME: 35 MINUTES

The secret to any great soup is a great stock. While there are many delicious vegetable stocks readily available at the supermarket, nothing will give you the depth and complexity of homemade stock. This recipe calls for the usual suspects, which you probably already have in your vegan cocina: tomatoes, onions, garlic, celery, mushrooms, and fresh herbs. Mushrooms give an incredible amount of richness to any stock. Swap buttons for other varieties for different flavors and intensities. The trick is to sweat the vegetables before simmering to develop the naturally sweet flavors.

1 tablespoon olive oil
2 onions, diced medium
2 large carrots, diced medium
4 celery stalks, diced medium
½ pound white button mushrooms, quartered
1 to 2 garlic cloves, smashed

2 tomatoes, diced
1 bay leaf
1 sprig fresh thyme
10 whole peppercorns
1 gallon water
Parsley stems (save the pretty green leaves for something else)

1. Heat the oil in a large stock pot on medium-low heat and add the onions, carrots, celery, mushrooms, garlic, and tomatoes. Cook the vegetables uncovered for 10 minutes, stirring occasionally. Be careful not to get too much color on them, as it can make the stock too dark, which would alter the color of anything you use the stock for.

2. Add the bay leaf, thyme, peppercorns, and water. Bring to a boil, reduce the heat, and simmer, uncovered, for 35 minutes.

3. Strain the stock through a colander and cool completely.

4. Store in the refrigerator in an airtight container for up to a week, or in the freezer for months.

COOKING TIP: Freezing stock in ice cube trays is a great way to store it if you only need a little at a time.

HANDMADE CORN TORTILLAS

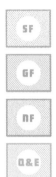

MAKES 12 TORTILLAS • PREP TIME: 20 MINUTES • COOK TIME: 12 MINUTES

Corn tortillas have been a staple of Mexican cuisine since Mesoamerican times, though they were known by a different name back then: tlaxcalli. *When the Spanish arrived in Mexico in the late 15th century and discovered these delightful flat corn breads made by the native Nahuatl people, they were renamed "tortilla." These quick handmade corn tortillas are so simple to make, you'll never need—or want—to buy the prepackaged variety again.*

2 cups corn masa flour
½ teaspoon salt
1½ cups warm water

1. Cut twenty-four 8-by-12-inch sheets of waxed paper for the tortilla press.

2. In a large bowl, mix together the corn masa flour and salt. Add the water and combine.

3. Divide the masa into 12 equal portions and form into football-shaped masa rolls.

4. Line the bottom of the tortilla press with a sheet of waxed paper and place one masa roll in the center of the press. Cover the roll with another piece of waxed paper. Press the masa into a thin disc. Remove the masa disc, still between the waxed paper sheets, and set aside. Repeat until all the rolls have been pressed.

5. If you don't have a tortilla press, don't stress. Line a cutting board with waxed paper, place a masa roll in the center, and cover with another piece of wax paper. Press the masa with a large, heavy hardcover book, such as a dictionary or encyclopedia.

6. Heat a large nonstick griddle or skillet on medium heat and lightly spray with nonstick cooking spray. Carefully peel the top sheet of waxed paper from a pressed masa. Place the disc directly onto the griddle (waxed paper facing up). Carefully peel the waxed paper from the masa, making sure not to tear the disc.

7. Cook for about 30 seconds on each side, or until the tortilla is evenly browned on both sides. Place the cooked tortillas in a tortilla warmer and serve.

COOKING TIP: Tortilla warmers are an essential part of any Mexican kitchen. They can keep tortillas warm, soft, and fresh for up to 1 hour. No tortilla warmer? No worries. Just loosely wrap the tortilla stack with a slightly moist kitchen towel and place them in a slow cooker set on low heat.

HANDMADE FLOUR TORTILLAS

MAKES 15 TO 20 TORTILLAS • PREP TIME: 5 MINUTES, PLUS 30 MINUTES RESTING TIME • COOK TIME: 25 MINUTES

It's hard to think of a more perfect comfort food than the flour tortilla. Originally derived from the native corn tortilla, flour tortillas were invented by Spanish Jews living in northern Mexico—including what is now Texas—because they didn't consider cornmeal to be kosher. This delicious flatbread led to the creation of the original burrito, and is now wildly popular across the world. Enjoy this foolproof recipe for anything from tacos to fajitas, or just rolled up and eaten on their own.

3 cups all-purpose flour, plus more for kneading and rolling
1 teaspoon salt
½ teaspoon baking powder
½ cup vegetable shortening
1¼ cups warm water

1. In a large mixing bowl, whisk together the flour, salt, and baking powder. Add the shortening and use your fingers to mix well.

2. Add the water and use your hands to combine and form the dough.

3. On a lightly floured surface, knead the dough for 4 to 5 minutes or until you have a nice smooth dough.

4. Divide the dough into 15 to 20 equal portions and roll into balls. Place the dough balls in the mixing bowl and cover with plastic wrap. Let the dough rest for 25 to 30 minutes.

5. Heat an ungreased griddle or skillet over medium-high heat.

6. On a lightly floured surface, use a rolling pin to roll out a portion of the dough into an even 6-inch to 8-inch disc.

7. Place the tortilla on the hot griddle for about 30 to 40 seconds. Flip the tortilla over and cook for another 30 to 40 seconds. Remove and wrap in a towel placed in a tortilla warmer. Roll and cook the remaining tortillas and stack them on top of each other in the tortilla warmer.

COOKING TIP: If you don't want to cook all the tortillas at once, roll each ball out into a disc and stack them on a large dinner plate with pieces of waxed paper between each disc. Wrap the dinner plate with plastic wrap and store in refrigerator for up to 3 days.

HANDMADE SOPES

SF

GF

NF

MAKES 8 SOPES • PREP TIME: 15 MINUTES • COOK TIME: 30 MINUTES

Sopes are delightful palm-size deep-dish corn cakes that originated in the northwestern Mexican city of Culiacán. The perfect sope is fried just right, so that the outside is crispy and the inside is still soft and doughy. Like Tlacoyo (page 106), the preparation method can seem complicated at first, but you'll get the hang of it quickly. Once you've perfected forming and frying the dough, you can pair your sopes with any number of delicious toppings. Serve as a hearty appetizer.

2 cups corn masa flour
½ teaspoon salt

1½ cups warm water
2 to 4 tablespoons canola oil

1. Cut 16 6-inch-square sheets of waxed paper for your tortilla press.

2. In a large bowl, mix the corn masa flour, salt, and warm water. Knead the dough until it is well combined. Divide the dough into eight pieces of the same size and form into balls.

3. Heat a small skillet over medium-high heat.

4. Line the bottom of the tortilla press with a sheet of waxed paper and place one masa roll in the center of the press. Cover the roll with another piece of waxed paper. Press the masa into a ½-inch-thick disc. Remove the masa disc, still between the waxed paper sheets, and set aside. Repeat until all the rolls have been pressed.

5. Place a masa disc on the dry, hot skillet. Cook each for 45 to 60 seconds, then flip and cook for another 45 to 60 seconds. Remove the disc from skillet and cover with a dry kitchen towel and allow to cool for about 60 seconds. Form the sopes by pinching up the edges with your fingers to create a pie shape. Be careful not to burn your fingers, as the disc will release hot steam when forming.

6. Repeat with the remaining seven discs of dough.

7. Heat the oil in a deeper skillet on medium heat. Place the sopes on the skillet and lightly fry them on both sides, about 30 to 45 seconds per side, or until golden brown. Remove from the heat and place on a paper towel–lined plate.

COOKING TIP: Fresh sopes should be served immediately. A common topping is refried beans, guacamole, and shredded lettuce.

CLASSIC GUACAMOLE

MAKES ABOUT 4 CUPS • PREP TIME: 5 MINUTES

While many claim to have the perfect "classic" guacamole recipe, the one thing I think we can all agree on is that we should always make a ton of it to have on hand. Avocado—the heart of guacamole—is a good source of potassium, B vitamins, and more. Spread guac on your favorite torta, plop some into a gringo taco, or toss it in a bowl as a standalone dip at your next party.

3 large, ripe Hass avocadoes, peeled and pitted
½ medium white onion, finely diced
1 small jalapeño chile, seeded and finely diced

1 large Roma tomato, seeded and diced
2 tablespoons chopped cilantro
Juice of 1 lime
½ teaspoon salt

1. In a large mixing bowl or molcajete, mash the avocados until they are mostly creamy, leaving some chunks.

2. Add the remaining ingredients and mix well. Serve fresh.

ORIGIN STORY: Fun to eat, fun to make, and fun to abbreviate, guacamole (guac!) has been around since the Aztecs' *āhuacamolli* hit the scene hundreds of years ago in what is now southern Mexico.

SWEET PEA SKINNY GUACAMOLE

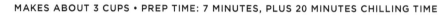

MAKES ABOUT 3 CUPS • PREP TIME: 7 MINUTES, PLUS 20 MINUTES CHILLING TIME

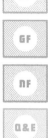

I love to run. I love to cook. I love guacamole. This skinny version of the already healthy and delicious traditional guacamole combines all three of those loves. Adding peas to the mix cuts some of the calories from the avocado and adds a protein punch that helps my body refuel after a run and gives me the energy I need to get back out there. Also, sometimes you just want to play with new flavors. This modern take on guac is a winner.

1 large, ripe Hass avocado, peeled and pitted
Juice of 1½ to 2 limes
½ teaspoon salt
2 cups fresh peas, or frozen and defrosted peas

½ medium white onion, finely diced
1 small jalapeño chile, seeded and finely diced
1 large Roma tomato, seeded and diced
2 tablespoons chopped fresh cilantro

1. In a large bowl, mash the avocado. Add the lime juice and salt and mix well.

2. In a small food processor or blender, process the peas until they are creamy. Add to the avocado mixture and combine.

3. Add the onion, jalapeño, tomato, and cilantro, and mix. Refrigerate for at least 20 minutes before serving.

SECRET INGREDIENT: Always use ripe avocados for guacamole. A ripe avocado is slightly soft when gently squeezed. Use a small paper bag to speed up the ripening process for unripe avocados. Place the avocado in the bag alongside a banana, apple, or tomato to trap their natural ethylene gas, which ripens the fruits. Close the bag and store on the countertop at room temperature for about up to 48 hours. Check for ripeness after 24 hours.

TOFU HUEVOS

SERVES 4 • PREP TIME: 5 MINUTES • COOK TIME: 10 TO 15 MINUTES

Tofu huevos are an essential ingredient for breakfast classics like Tofu Huevos Rancheros (page 35), Migas (page 38), and all great Breakfast Burritos (page 128). The key to making the perfect tofu huevos is to keep them simple and versatile, so their breakfast counterparts can be the star of the dish. I recommend cooking the turmeric for a couple of minutes before tossing the tofu and spices into the skillet, to help reduce its bitterness.

1 tablespoon canola oil
½ teaspoon ground turmeric
1 (1-pound) package silken
    tofu, drained

½ teaspoon onion powder
¼ teaspoon garlic powder
¼ teaspoon ground cumin
½ teaspoon salt

1. In a large skillet, heat the oil on low heat and cook the turmeric for 2 minutes.

2. Turn up the heat to medium, add the tofu, and break into a crumble with a spoon. Add the onion powder, garlic powder, cumin, and salt. Scramble.

3. Cook for 5 to 10 minutes, stirring occasionally.

SIMPLE SWAP: Try replacing the salt with ¼ teaspoon of black Himalayan salt (kala namak) for a slightly eggier flavor. If you're using black salt, use half the amount because it's saltier.

SEARED CHICKEN-STYLE SETAS

SERVES 4 TO 6 • PREP TIME: 5 MINUTES, PLUS 1 TO 4 HOURS MARINATING TIME •
COOK TIME: 15 MINUTES

The oyster mushroom is, hands down, my favorite mushroom. I was first introduced to the flavorful fungi at a tapas bar in northwest Spain during a summer trip to visit my brother. The dish was called Setas al Ajillo, and it consisted of three simple ingredients: olive oil, garlic, and oyster mushrooms. The modest dish blew me away, and I spent much of the summer cooking with oyster mushrooms and exploring their vast versatility. I now use oyster mushrooms for any dish that calls for chicken, and any way I choose to cook them, they don't disappoint. This fast-seared recipe truly showcases the oyster mushroom's amazing ability to mimic marinated, seared chicken.

3 tablespoons olive oil
3 to 4 tablespoons spice blend or rub
    of your choice
2 pounds fresh oyster mushrooms

1. In a large bowl, mix the olive oil and seasonings to form a thick paste. Rub into the mushrooms and marinate for 1 to 4 hours.

2. Preheat a cast-iron skillet on medium-high heat and add the mushrooms and the marinade. Press the mushrooms with a second cast-iron skillet or a steak-weight grill press. Both pans will be very hot, so be extremely careful not to burn yourself or the mushrooms.

3. Sear for about 4 to 5 minutes, then turn the mushrooms over and press again. Sear for another 4 to 5 minutes.

4. Reduce the heat to medium and cook for about 5 more minutes, stirring occasionally.

5. Remove the mushrooms from the pan and let rest for 2 to 3 minutes before slicing. They should have a very nice char to them, but be soft and cooked through on the inside.

COOKING TIP: Do make sure to wear heat-resistant gloves and have plenty of ventilation when using this method of preparation. When searing, the smokiness and spiciness can get quite intense, particularly in small spaces.

MEXICAN SEASONED SEITAN

SERVES 10 • PREP TIME: 15 MINUTES • COOK TIME: 1 TO 1½ HOURS

Where's the meat? Seitan, otherwise known as wheat meat, is the every-thing meat. Throughout this book you will find that seasoned seitan is the foundation for the meats used in a wide variety of beefy dishes. What I love about seitan is that it is incredibly versatile. It can be cut into steaks or strips to be seared or grilled. It can also be cut into chunks and stewed. Crispy or tender, seitan delivers. Seitan can be seasoned so many differ-ent ways, but for this batch we'll season it so it will work in nearly any Mexican-inspired recipe.

2 cups vital wheat gluten
2 teaspoons ground cumin
2 teaspoons chili powder
2 teaspoons granulated garlic
1 teaspoon freshly ground black pepper

2 cups warm water
2 quarts Homemade Vegetable
   Stock (page 231)
3 tablespoons soy sauce or Bragg
   liquid aminos

1. Add the vital wheat gluten, cumin, chili powder, garlic, and pepper to a large mix-ing bowl and combine with a fork.

2. Add the warm water and continue mixing with a fork.

3. Knead the dough by hand about 5 or 6 times to toughen up the mixture and make it more elastic.

4. In a large soup pot, bring the Homemade Vegetable Stock and soy sauce to a boil.

5. Stretch out the dough ball to about 1½ to 2 inches thick. Cut it into 3-inch squares and place the squares in the boil-ing liquid. Restretching will be required, as the dough will be very springy.

6. Cook for 1 to 1½ hours, keeping a con-stant simmer in the pot.

7. Remove the seitan from the pot and drain.

8. Seitan can be stored in an airtight con-tainer in the refrigerator for 1 week.

COOKING TIP: For a different texture, you can bake the dough instead of simmer-ing it. Roll the dough into a log, wrap in foil, and bake in the oven at 325°F for 45 minutes. Turn the log over and bake for another 45 minutes. Done!

GREEN SEITAN CHORIZO

MAKES 8 SAUSAGES • PREP TIME: 15 MINUTES • COOK TIME: 45 TO 60 MINUTES

The city of Toluca, known as "La Bella" for its beautiful 19th-century colonial architecture, is the capital of the State of Mexico. It's also unofficially known as the chorizo capital of the country. Spicy green chile–infused seitan sausage is my salute to the chorizo capital. You can eat them right out of the steamer if you like, but a nice sear or some time on the grill can make these so wonderful. This recipe takes a little work, so make a batch and use it in a few different dishes.

2 tablespoons olive oil
½ white onion, minced
1 poblano chile, seeded and minced
2 serrano chiles, seeded and minced
4 garlic cloves, minced
1 (4-ounce) can hot roasted green chiles
½ cup canned pinto beans, drained and mashed well
3 tablespoons apple cider vinegar
Juice of 2 limes
2 cups vital wheat gluten

¼ cup nutritional yeast
2 tablespoons ground cumin
1 teaspoon onion powder
1 tablespoon spirulina powder or spinach powder (optional)
2 teaspoons dried Mexican oregano
2 teaspoons salt
1 teaspoon ground coriander
1 teaspoon freshly ground black pepper
2 cups Homemade Vegetable Stock (page 231)
Nonstick cooking spray

1. Heat the olive oil in a large pan and sauté the onion, poblano and serrano chiles, and garlic on medium heat for 5 minutes. Add the canned green chiles, mashed pinto beans, vinegar, and lime juice, and heat through. Remove from the heat.

2. In a large bowl, mix the vital wheat gluten, nutritional yeast, cumin, onion powder, spirulina or spinach powder (if using), oregano, salt, coriander, and black pepper with a whisk. Fold in the cooked chiles and beans. Pour in the Homemade Vegetable Stock and mix well with your hands, mashing and kneading the dough 5 or 6 times.

3. Spread out the seitan dough on a cutting board and cut into eight even pieces.

4. Lightly spray eight pieces of 8-by-6-inch aluminum foil with nonstick cooking spray.

5. Roll a piece of seitan dough in your hand and shape into a 6-inch long, 1-inch-thick sausage. Place the sausage in a foil wrapper, roll the foil around the sausage, twist up the ends, and fold them in.

6. Put about 2 inches of water in a large, deep steaming pot. Add a steamer basket, making sure the water line is below the basket. Place the sausages in the steamer basket in a row; if you need more room, stack them at right angles, like logs on a fire. You can also cook them in separate batches, if needed. Just make sure to leave room for the steam to move between the sausages and around the pot.

7. Cover and steam for about 45 to 60 minutes, adding more water to the pot as needed.

8. Remove the sausages from the heat and let cool. Unwrap when the sausages are cool enough to touch.

COOKING TIP: Be sure to wrap the sausages up tightly in the foil. They will swell when they cook, and you don't want them to bust loose of the foil. It makes a mess, and the sausages will not be as dense.

GARBANZORIZO

SERVES 4 • PREP TIME: 10 MINUTES • COOK TIME: 10 TO 15 MINUTES

Mexican chorizo is an intensely spiced sausage that's typically made with pork, vinegar, and variety of herbs, spices, and chiles. Earlier this year, I did a cooking demo for a popular morning television show in Mexico, where I featured a prototype of my now-famous Garbanzorizo recipe. The segment was recorded at a coworking space in the hip Roma neighborhood of Mexico City, and the aroma had flocks of workers crowding the set as soon as we wrapped up. They devoured it. This recipe calls for some unlikely characters, like ground cloves and sun-dried tomatoes. I've used both dry and oil-packed (in a jar) sun-dried tomatoes for this recipe, and they both work well. If you're using oil-packed sun-dried tomatoes, I recommend patting off some of the oil before chopping.

1½ tablespoons olive oil
½ cup yellow onion, finely diced
¼ teaspoon salt
4 garlic cloves, minced
½ teaspoon ground cumin
¼ teaspoon dried thyme
½ teaspoon dried Mexican oregano
¼ teaspoon freshly ground
   black pepper
¼ teaspoon ground cinnamon
⅛ teaspoon ground cloves

1 teaspoon ground coriander
½ teaspoon paprika
½ teaspoon chipotle powder
1 teaspoon chili powder
2½ tablespoons sun-dried tomatoes,
   finely chopped
1 (15-ounce) can chickpeas, drained
   and rinsed
1 teaspoon tamari
2 teaspoons apple cider vinegar

1. In a large pan, heat the oil at medium-high heat. Add the onion and salt and sauté for 4 to 5 minutes, or until the onion is nearly translucent. Add the garlic and stir together.

2. Add the cumin, thyme, oregano, pepper, cinnamon, cloves, coriander, paprika, chipotle and chili powders, and the chopped sun-dried tomatoes. Mix well.

3. Add the chickpeas, tamari, and vinegar, and toss until combined.

4. Mash the mixture lightly until the chickpeas are crumbly. Mix well and cook for 5 to 7 more minutes, stirring occasionally.

ORIGIN STORY: In 2013, the United Nations declared that 2016 would be the international year of pulses—legumes that grow inside pods. I had been experimenting with my favorite pulse, the chickpea, and a variety of spices to emulate Grandma's handmade Mexican chorizo. You can find soy-based versions at most US grocery stores, but I think you'll find my Garbanzorizo recipe to be more versatile. Just trust that you're getting an authentic taste of Grandma's home cooking.

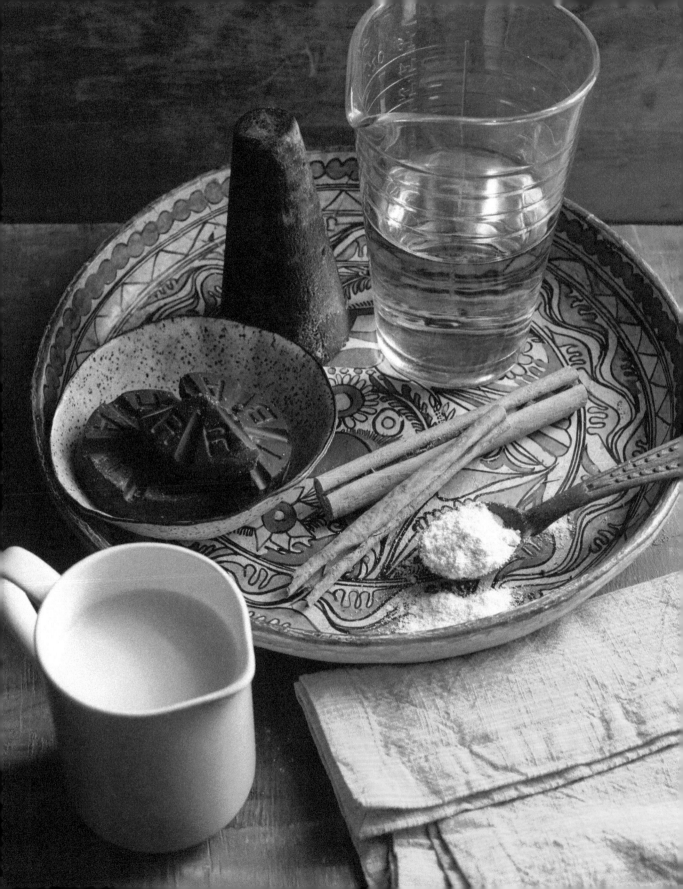

Resources

Food Products

It's never been easier—or tastier—to eat vegan. There are delicious plant-based alternatives to virtually every animal product, from milks and mayos to meats, cheeses, and eggs. Here are some of my favorite easy-to-find products. For all of them, their website will help you find local and online stores that sell their products.

JUST MAYO Just Mayo is an egg-free mayo made by Hampton Creek. It comes in a variety of flavors, including original, garlic, chipotle, and Sriracha. What replaces the egg in this completely cholesterol-free mayo is a specific variety of the Canadian field pea. You can find Just Mayo at most major supermarkets and online.

DAIYA DELICIOUSLY DAIRY FREE Lots of recipes in this cookbook call for vegan shredded cheese, and for most of them, I use Daiya mozzarella or Cheddar–style shreds because of their wonderful melt-ability. Daiya is a great option for anyone with sensitivities to gluten, soy, or nuts, because their products contain none of those things. You can find Daiya brand shreds and other dairy-free products in most health food markets and many well-stocked grocery stores.

FOLLOW YOUR HEART VEGAN GOURMET Vegan Gourmet by Follow Your Heart offers a variety of dairy alternatives, including mild-flavored shreds that melt perfectly and cream cheeses that make wonderfully flaky empanadas. Their products are available at most health food stores and well-stocked grocers.

Meat Alternatives

Most of the meaty recipes in this book feature my homemade Mexican Seasoned Seitan (page 239), texturized vegetable protein (TVP), or versatile fruits and veggies that mimic meaty textures. I strongly encourage you to try those first. But if you're pressed for time, there are so many prepackaged vegan meats on the market you can use. Here are some of my favorites.

GARDEIN The name combines the words *garden* and *protein*. Gardein makes a wide assortment of plant-based meats, like Crabless Cakes, which can be used for my Baja Burritos (page 127), and Chick'n Strips that can be used in place of oyster mushrooms for Enmoladas Verdes with Seared Chicken-Style Setas (page 238). Gardein products can be found at any health food store and many major supermarkets.

BEYOND MEAT I always have a package of Beyond Meat Beefy Crumbles in my freezer to speed up meals like Picadillo (page 63) and to throw in a pot of Sopa de Fideo (page 57) for a heartier noodle bowl. The company's Beyond Chicken–Lightly Seasoned Strips work really well in saucy dishes and stews. For a chicken-style pozole, I simply use my Seafood-Style Pozole recipe (page 61) and replace the dulse flakes and palm hearts with half a package of seasoned strips. You can find Beyond Meat products at most health food stores and many well-stocked grocery stores.

UPTON'S NATURALS Upton's Naturals makes cooked, shredded jackfruit that comes in a vacuum pouch-sealed pouch. It's available natural in three flavors, including Chili Lime Carnitas. They also make five flavors of seitan, including Chorizo and Bacon. Their products can be found at any health food store and many major supermarkets.

Get Online

WWW.HAPPYCOW.NET Happy Cow is an essential website and app for any traveling vegan. No matter where you are in the world, Happy Cow will direct you to nearest vegan-friendly health food stores, supermarkets, and restaurants. Happy Cow pointed me to what are now some of favorite vegan Latin restaurants: like Vspot in New York City; Choices Café in Miami; Vegeria in San Antonio; El Palote in Dallas; La Oveja Verde in Monterrey, Mexico; and Por Siempre Vegana Taqueria and Forever Vegano in Mexico City.

WWW.HUMANESOCIETY.ORG The Humane Society of the United States promotes eating with conscience and embracing the Three Rs: reducing the consumption of meat and other animal-based foods; refining the diet by avoiding products from the worst production systems; and replacing meat and other animal-based foods in the diet with plant-based foods. For a free *Guide to Meat-free Meals* and to learn more about the benefits of a plant-powered diet, go to HumaneSociety.org/Meatfree. You'll also find hundreds of delicious meat-free recipes that range from Mexican to Italian to American fare, and more.

Go Shopping

WWW.MEXGROCER.COM All major US cities have at least one Latin market, where you can find essential ingredients like chiles, corn flour, and Mexican chocolate. But if you're in a smaller city or looking for some of those harder-to-find ingredients like huitlacoche and banana leaves, I suggest heading to MexGrocer.com for everything from dried goods to fresh produce to Mexican kitchen tools.

WWW.RABBITFOODGROCERY.COM Rabbit Food Grocery offers only vegan items, including grocery staples, body care products, household supplies, clothing, and gifts.

WWW.VEGANESSENTIALS.COM This huge site has more than 2,000 vegan items, including cosmetics, body care, clothing, shoes, accessories, food, beverages, books, and vitamins.

Measurement Conversions

Volume Equivalents (Liquid)

US STANDARD	US STANDARD (OUNCES)	METRIC (APPROXIMATE)
2 tablespoons	1 fl. oz.	30 mL
¼ cup	2 fl. oz.	60 mL
½ cup	4 fl. oz.	120 mL
1 cup	8 fl. oz.	240 mL
1½ cups	12 fl. oz.	355 mL
2 cups or 1 pint	16 fl. oz.	475 mL
4 cups or 1 quart	32 fl. oz.	1 L
1 gallon	128 fl. oz.	4 L

Oven Temperatures

FAHRENHEIT (F)	CELSIUS (C) (APPROXIMATE)
250°F	120°C
300°F	150°C
325°F	165°C
350°F	180°C
375°F	190°C
400°F	200°C
425°F	220°C
450°F	230°C

Volume Equivalents (Dry)

US STANDARD	METRIC (APPROXIMATE)
⅛ teaspoon	0.5 mL
¼ teaspoon	1 mL
½ teaspoon	2 mL
¾ teaspoon	4 mL
1 teaspoon	5 mL
1 tablespoon	15 mL
¼ cup	59 mL
⅓ cup	79 mL
½ cup	118 mL
⅔ cup	156 mL
¾ cup	177 mL
1 cup	235 mL
2 cups or 1 pint	475 mL
3 cups	700 mL
4 cups or 1 quart	1 L

Weight Equivalents

US STANDARD	METRIC (APPROXIMATE)
½ ounce	15 g
1 ounce	30 g
2 ounces	60 g
4 ounces	115 g
8 ounces	225 g
12 ounces	340 g
16 ounces or 1 pound	455 g

Index

Acknowledgments

First and foremost, I want to thank my grandma, Soledad, for all the incredible support she has shown me over the years and for teaching me to be proud of who I am and where I came from. I also want to thank my mom and dad, Emma and Juan Miguel, who taught me to work hard and never give up on what I believe in.

To my brother and sister-in-law, Michael and Erica: Thank you for your endless encouragement and for bringing me the greatest joy of my life—my sweet nephew Sammy.

To Ari: Thank you, *hermano*, for always inspiring me—and enabling me—to take my yoga practice beyond the mat.

To Sara at Spiral Diner & Bakery: Thank you for taking a chance on a nerdy music teacher that one special summer.

John: You're a rock star. I can't thank you enough, brother, for your incredible help and mentorship throughout this entire process.

Ethan, Irene, Jamey, Josh, Kristie, Lisa, Mark, Paul, and Sara: Your friendship means the world to me.

And a huge thanks to all my friends and colleagues at the Humane Society of the United States for their amazing support and for their tireless work to defend animals.

About the Author

EDDIE GARZA is Senior Manager of Food & Nutrition for the Humane Society of the United States and is a leading figure in the movement to reform food systems in Latino communities. Garza and his work have been featured by a wide variety of media outlets in the United States and Mexico, including CNN, Fox News Latino, TV Azteca, Latin Times, Telemundo, and Univision.

Garza has collaborated with some of the nation's most influential school districts and higher education institutions to develop and implement innovative plant-based meal programs, and has conducted culinary trainings and ideations for major hospitals, restaurant groups, culinary schools, and public school systems in regions with large Hispanic populations.

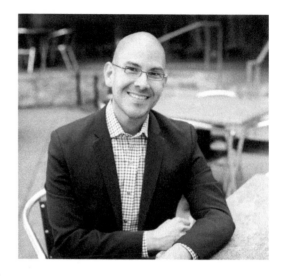

He's a sought-after speaker, culinary coach, published writer, and thought leader on issues related to Latino health, and has lectured and presented at top universities, public school forums, and major conferences, including South by Southwest in Austin and ExpoSer in Mexico City.

CPSIA information can be obtained
at www.ICGtesting.com
Printed in the USA
LVHW070833061020
667891LV00001BA/1